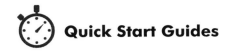 **Quick Start Guides**

THE VEGAN 15 MINUTE
COOKBOOK

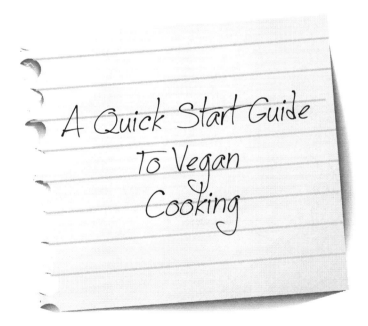

A Quick Start Guide To Vegan Cooking

Over 100 Simple And Delicious Vegan Recipes For Everyone

First published in 2018 by Erin Rose Publishing

Text and illustration copyright © 2018 Erin Rose Publishing

Design: Julie Anson

ISBN: 978-1-911492-21-4

A CIP record for this book is available from the British Library.

DISCLAIMER: This book is for informational purposes only and not intended as a substitute for the medical advice, diagnosis or treatment of a physician or qualified healthcare provider. The reader should consult a physician before undertaking a new health care regime and in all matters relating to his/her health, and particularly with respect to any symptoms that may require diagnosis or medical attention.

While every care has been taken in compiling the recipes for this book we cannot accept responsibility for any problems which arise as a result of preparing one of the recipes. The author and publisher disclaim responsibility for any adverse effects that may arise from the use or application of the recipes in this book. Some of the recipes in this book include nuts or other allergens. If you have an allergy it's important to avoid these.

CONTENTS

Recipes

INTRODUCTION

Whether you are starting out on a vegan diet or if you are looking for new, quick and tasty recipes which can be cooked in 15 minutes, you need to look no further. Eating a vegan diet has never been easier!

In this book there are over 100 delicious recipes to make vegan cooking fast and easy, ideal for when you are short on time. When starting a vegan diet, it's important to know what you can and can't eat and to understand what substitutions you can make to prevent the temptation of eating fast junk food, albeit vegan, when you aren't sure what else to eat. A vegan diet will provide you with an abundance of vitamins, minerals, antioxidants and micro-nutrients and you'll be heaping delicious flavours and textures together, giving your plenty of variety and helping you feel sated.

The recipes in the Quick Start Guide are full of wholefoods and fresh ingredients, avoiding the use of foods which are hard to come by, as everything is available in most supermarkets. Vegan cooking really doesn't have to feel limiting.

Veganism is increasing and is more than just a trend. It is a change of lifestyle and it's here to stay! The worldwide growth of veganism shows it is a fast growing lifestyle, avoiding the consumption of animal products for a more ethical approach, benefitting our health, the welfare of animals and the environment. A vegan diet is now one of the most popular diets in the world and it's growing fast.

For the individual, eating a vegan diet means you will be eating more fresh, healthy food then before, increasing your nutrient intake, having more energy, feeling lighter, less bloating and indigestion and subsequently shedding excess weight. And the bonus is that vegan food tastes delicious.

If you are ready to experience the benefits and willing to try exciting new recipes, read on!

Why Go Vegan?

There are several reasons why people chose a vegan diet. Firstly, animal welfare. Sometimes people don't like to think about it but by following a vegan diet you make the personal choice to make an impact to reduce the suffering of animals. Vegans strongly believe that the animal's right to life is a priority and the prevention of cruelty, harm and unnecessary suffering. Respecting the animal's right to life also extends to avoiding products such as cosmetics, cleaning products and clothing which are not vegan.

Eating a vegan diet can be inexpensive and save you money on your grocery bill too. Vegan forms of protein are less expensive than animal products so it benefits your purse.

Healthy weight loss is a proven benefit of a balanced vegan diet, partly because the food is less calorific and can therefore reduce your Body Mass Index. A large plate of plant based food can contain far less calories than an average portion of a meat based meal. It's much more than just eating your 5 portions of fruit and veg a day. You pack in high nutrient foods and plenty of them.

A vegan diet is high in essential nutrients and vitamins like potassium, magnesium, vitamin C, antioxidants and fibre. You can still eat plenty of protein like, nuts, seeds, grains and legumes which contain plenty of amino acids, necessary for a healthy body. Iron is available in broccoli, green leafy vegetables, grains and dried fruit like raisins and apricots. Chemicals, hormones and salt in meat, especially processed meat, are linked to cardiovascular disease, diabetes and cancer.

The meat industry is the third largest contributor to climate change. Raising livestock for food involves transportation which produces emissions which have a negative impact on the environment. The farming of vast numbers of cattle requires vast fuel resources, water and land which is used for animal feed crops. So much of the meat in our supply is wasted and a reduction in meat production can help reduce greenhouse gas.

What Can I Eat?

Foods To Avoid

Avoid all animal products including the following:

- Beef
- Chicken
- Pork
- Turkey
- Lamb
- Fowl
- Fish
- Venison
- Veal
- Animal Fat

- Eggs
- Milk
- Cream
- Cheese
- Yogurt
- Crème Fraîche
- Fromage Frais
- Butter
- Honey
- Gelatine

Foods You Can Eat

Fruits & Vegetables

- Avocados
- Aubergine (Eggplant)
- Broccoli
- Beetroot
- Brussels Sprouts
- Cauliflower
- Capers
- Cabbage
- Celeriac
- Celery
- Courgette (Zucchini)
- Cucumber
- Carrots
- Garlic
- Kale
- Lettuce
- Fennel
- Mushrooms
- Onions
- Marrow
- Peppers

- Parsnip
- Peas
- Potatoes
- Radishes
- Rocket (Arugula)
- Seaweeds like nori and dulse
- Spring Onions (Scallions)
- Shallots
- Soya
- Spinach
- Sweet Potatoes
- Swede
- Tomatoes
- Turnip
- Apples
- Bananas
- Blackberries
- Blueberries
- Grapefruit
- Kiwi Fruit
- Lemons
- Limes

- Mango
- Oranges
- Pineapple
- Raspberries
- Redcurrants
- Lychees
- Peaches
- Pears
- Persimmon
- Nectarines
- Strawberries

Dried fruit

- Raisins
- Cranberries
- Currants
- Dates
- Bananas
- Apples
- Figs
- Sultanas
- Apricots
- Prunes

Herbs & Spices

- Parsley
- Basil
- Bay Leaves
- Oregano
- Thyme
- Chives
- Cardamom Seeds
- Coriander (Cilantro)
- Lemon Balm
- Tarragon
- Dill
- Sage
- Cumin
- Turmeric
- Cayenne Pepper
- Mustard
- Ginger
- Chilli
- Nutmeg
- Allspice
- Star Anise
- Cinnamon
- Paprika
- Asafoetida

Pulses, Nuts & Seeds

- Brazil Nuts
- Almonds
- Coconuts
- Walnuts
- Pecans
- Pine Nuts
- Pistachios
- Hazelnuts
- Peanuts
- Cashew Nuts
- Soybeans (Edamame)
- Black Beans
- Kidney Beans
- Cannellini Beans
- Haricot Beans
- Kidney Beans
- Chickpeas (Garbanzo Beans)
- Aduki Beans
- Pinto Beans
- Lentils
- Peas
- Chia Seeds
- Pumpkin Seeds

- Hemp Seeds
- Flaxseeds (Linseeds)
- Poppy Seeds
- Sesame Seeds
- Sunflower Seeds
- All nut butters, nut milks and nut oils.

Grains & Cereals

- Rice
- Quinoa
- Buckwheat
- Oats
- Corn
- Amaranth
- Polenta
- Millet
- Wheat
- Barley
- Rye
- Bulgur Wheat
- Couscous

Soya Products

- Tofu
- Soya Milk

- Soya Yogurt
- Soya Cheese
- Soya Protein
- Tempeh
- Miso

Additional

- Dairy-Free Dark Chocolate, Cacao Nibs or 100% Cocoa Powder
- Agave Nectar
- Maple Syrup
- Blackstrap Molasses
- Golden Syrup
- Sugar
- Tahini
- Nut Butters: like peanut butter, cashew butter and almond butter
- Nutritional Yeast
- Olive Oil
- Coconut Oil
- Vanilla Extract, Vanilla Pods
- Vinegar
- Soy Sauce
- Tabasco Sauce
- Coconut Cream/Coconut Milk

Tips For Fast Vegan Cooking

Making healthy vegan cooking as simple as possible is a must for anyone with a busy lifestyle – which is most of us. We want you to have the time to cook delicious dishes without having to spend hours in the kitchen.

Selecting your store-cupboard essentials and keeping a stock of basic ingredients will ensure you have what you need to prepare and cook if you have limited time.

You can make a shopping list in advance and plan your meals to make the most of the food you have prepared. For instance, if you make a tray of roast vegetables, or a big pot of chilli beans larger than you need, you can keep them in the fridge so that you have plenty of leftovers to make Buddha bowls. Make some extra rice or quinoa and keep it in the fridge then you can assemble the ingredients with your favourite dressing, guacamole or hummus and you have a tasty meal ready in only a few minutes. Or you can freeze your leftovers and have a stock of homemade meals and treats readily available if you don't have time to shop or if you need an ingredient to make soups or smoothies.

Packs of frozen fruit are an absolute winner! They are frozen when they are fresh, ripe and in peak condition and when it comes to avocados it saves time and waste when you don't have to remove black bits or cut in and find it's either over or under ripe. Another benefit of using frozen fruit is that you don't have to add ice cubes to have a cold smoothie.

Vegetables can be bought pre-prepared but here the taste difference is sometimes tangible as it can be drying out and lacking nutrients. It'll depend on how fresh it is on the supermarket shelf to begin with and if you can use it the same day, or within 2 days, it could be a good option. To reduce cooking time, chop vegetables into smaller pieces.

Adjust recipes and substitute ingredients to what you have in the fridge, for instance if a recipe asks for lettuce but you've run out, you can use a handful of fresh spinach leaves from the bag in the fridge. It'll cut down on waste and reduce any spoiling vegetable waste.

If you are taking lunches to work, mason jars are a great way of keeping salads fresh and they prevent them from being tossed around and becoming unappetising looking before you eat them. You can add layers of ingredients to mason jars, starting with the heaviest at the bottom and light leaves at the top – the dressing can be added either in the bottom layer if you don't want it coating everything just yet, or drizzled over the top. Remember to keep in the fridge until ready to use.

You can make use of ingredients like jars of chopped garlic, ginger and chilli and use a small amount of these to replace the fresh variety if you wish to save yourself more time.

You can multiply the quantities of recipes to ensure you have a batch to freeze, especially when it comes to soups and chillies.

Make a list of your store cupboard essentials and be sure to include plenty of tins of beans, lentils, tinned tomatoes, coconut milk, sweetcorn, tomato purée and/or passata.

A selection of dried spices will keep really well and you can jazz up the flavour of simple dishes by using them. Dried herbs are also useful and you'll find you need less of the dried version than you do of fresh herbs however the scent and flavour of fresh herbs is preferable, so herbs growing on the windowsill are a great option.

Always check with your medical advisor or doctor before embarking on any radical dietary changes, especially if you suffer from any medication condition, to ensure that it is safe and appropriate for you to do so.

Vegan Substitutes

If you are new to vegan cooking it may take a little getting used to and you may wish to experiment to find your favourite ingredients. Due to demand, there are now more vegan foodstuffs on offer at the supermarket, ranging from vegan cheese, to soya cream and cashew milk. In terms of desired flavour and texture, these may be an acquired taste, but they will expand your meal variety.

Finding a plant-based milk is probably the most important. Almond milk is one of the most popular. It does not have a particularly strong flavour and is a good 'milky' consistency without being too thin. Soya milk is still popular and like almond milk is available sweetened or unsweetened. The range of plant milks available is still expanding. Once you have found plant-based milks you like, you can stock up as they keep well.

As an egg replacement in recipes which require binding, you can use chickpea flour (garbanzo bean flour/gram flour), or ground flaxseeds (linseeds). You could also use scrambled tofu as a substitute for scrambled egg.

Vegetable bouillon is a suitable replacement for meat stocks and this is another great store cupboard food.

Try coconut yogurt or soya yogurt as an alternative to dairy yogurt. Coconut yogurt is particularly delicious although it usually isn't cheap. These are available in the chilled section at the supermarket.

There are many solutions to not having butter. You can use peanut butter, cashew butter, almond butter, olive oil, coconut oil and mixed seed butter (this is so good!). Another possibility is margarine although you will need to check the labelling to make sure it is vegan. The drawback with margarines is that they can contain unhealthy hydrogenated fats.

Maple syrup, molasses, brown rice syrup and agave nectar can be used in place of honey. Dates can be added to recipes and give a delicious toffee flavour plus they contain fibre which slows down the sugar absorption.

Try not to over indulge on sweet things as too much sugar is never a good thing and can leave you with cravings. Some people choose to avoid cane sugar as some brands use animal bone char in the refining process.

Good quality chocolate is good for you and you don't have to give it up. There are dairy-free chocolates available plus 100% cocoa powder and cacao nibs.

Tofu is a nutritious protein which can be added to many dishes. It can be kept in the fridge or freezer in various forms like mince, blocks of smoked tofu and silken tofu for desserts. Again, you may need to experiment to find one you like.

Avoiding eating meat may be the greatest challenge for some. There are plenty of ready-made alternatives on the market including bacon, cheese, burgers, meat and meat balls which are all suitable for vegans. However, to avoid too many additives in your food, home-cooked meals are still better.

Reading the Labels

Some products carry the 'suitable for vegans' logo, however this is not currently on all products and there are ready-made foods available to you which don't contain animal derived ingredients. If you wish to be sure a product is vegan it is worth checking the labels. Even products which appear to be free from animal products can contain non-vegan ingredients, often in the form of a dairy product. Below is a list of terms you may find on the package labels to help you decipher if it is a true vegan product. Some of these are obvious and others less so. It is also worth checking that your plant milk does not have whey added to it!

- **Animal Fats**
- **Beef Extract**
- **Beef Stock**
- **Beeswax**
- **Butter Fat**
- **Butter Oil**
- **Butter Ester**
- **Butter Milk**
- **Bone Char**
- **Bone Phosphate**
- **Carmine**
- **Casein**
- **Casein Hydrolysate**
- **Caseinates**
- **Curds**

- **Ghee**
- **Gelling Agent**
- **Lactose**
- **Lactalbumin**
- **Lactoferrin**
- **Lactose**
- **Lactulose**
- **Lactitol**
- **L-Cysteine**
- **Milk Protein Hydrolysate**
- **Whey**
- **Whey Protein Hydrolysate**
- **Albumen**
- **Dried Egg**
- **Egg Solids**

- Mayonnaise
- Modified Milk
- Meringue
- Cochineal
- Aspic
- Tallow
- Collagen
- Elastin
- Cod Liver Oil
- Fish Oil
- Gelatine
- Rennet
- Pepsin
- Shellac

E numbers which are derived from animal products are;

- E901
- E120
- E966
- E441
- E542
- E904
- E910
- E920
- E921

Recipes

BREAKFAST

Hot Chocolate & Banana Smoothie Bowl

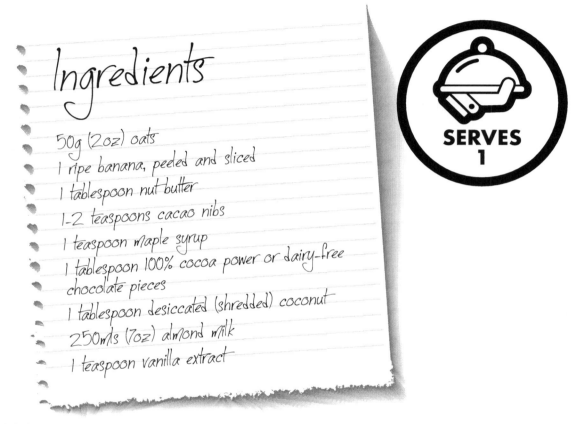

Ingredients

50g (2oz) oats

1 ripe banana, peeled and sliced

1 tablespoon nut butter

1-2 teaspoons cacao nibs

1 teaspoon maple syrup

1 tablespoon 100% cocoa power or dairy-free chocolate pieces

1 tablespoon desiccated (shredded) coconut

250mls (7oz) almond milk

1 teaspoon vanilla extract

SERVES 1

Method

Place all of the ingredients apart from the cacao nibs, banana and coconut into a food processor or smoothie maker and blitz until smooth. Pour the smoothie into a saucepan and warm it gently. Transfer it to a serving bowl. Lay the banana slices down one side and add a little heap of coconut at the edge. You can also garnish it with cacao nibs if you wish. If you'd prefer your smoothie bowl cold just skip warming it up and garnish it before serving.

Blueberry, Cashew & Coconut Smoothie Bowl

Ingredients

100g (3½ oz) blueberries, fresh or frozen

50g (2oz) desiccated (shredded) coconut

1 large banana

1 tablespoon cashew nuts, chopped

1 tablespoon chia seeds

100mls (3½ fl oz) almond milk or other plant milk

SERVES 1

Method

Place all of the ingredients, apart from the cashews, chia seeds and a few blueberries into a food processor or smoothie maker and process until smooth. Transfer the smoothie to a serving bowl. Add little heaps of chopped cashews, chia seeds and a few blueberries. You can be as creative as you like with smoothie bowl. Experiment with different types of fruit and remember not to add water to the food processor so that your smoothie base is nice and thick. You can add various nuts, seeds, berries and cacao nibs – or even add matcha or spirulina for an energy boost.

Strawberry & Avocado Smoothie

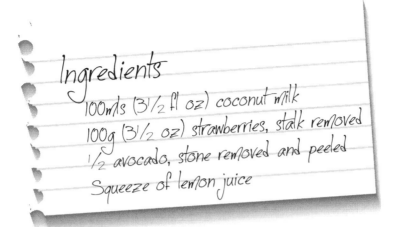

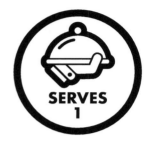

SERVES
1

Ingredients
100mls (3½ fl oz) coconut milk
100g (3½ oz) strawberries, stalk removed
½ avocado, stone removed and peeled
Squeeze of lemon juice

Method

Toss all of the ingredients into a food processor and blitz until smooth and creamy. You can add a little water if you like it less thick.

Apple, Pear and Spinach Smoothie

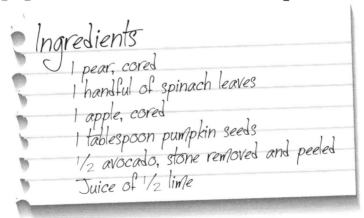

SERVES
1

Ingredients
1 pear, cored
1 handful of spinach leaves
1 apple, cored
1 tablespoon pumpkin seeds
½ avocado, stone removed and peeled
Juice of ½ lime

Method

Put all the ingredients into a blender with just enough water to cover the ingredients. Blitz until smooth. You can add more lime juice for extra zing.

Carrot, Apple & Ginger Smoothie

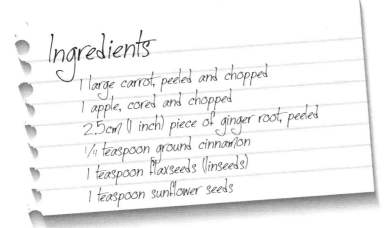

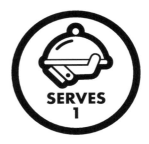

SERVES 1

Ingredients
1 large carrot, peeled and chopped
1 apple, cored and chopped
2.5cm (1 inch) piece of ginger root, peeled
1/4 teaspoon ground cinnamon
1 teaspoon flaxseeds (linseeds)
1 teaspoon sunflower seeds

Method

Place all of the ingredients into a blender with just enough water to cover them and blitz until smooth. If your blender doesn't process seeds or nuts you can add in the ground version.

Kiwi Salad Shots

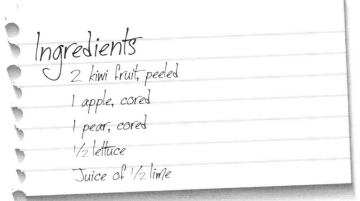

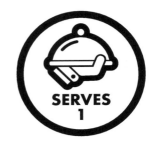

SERVES 1

Ingredients
2 kiwi fruit, peeled
1 apple, cored
1 pear, cored
1/2 lettuce
Juice of 1/2 lime

Method

Place the ingredients into a food processor and add just enough water to cover them and blitz until smooth. Pour the liquid into a glass bottle. Store it in the fridge, ready for you to have fresh shots throughout the day or you can simply drink it all straight away.

Creamy Peach Smoothie

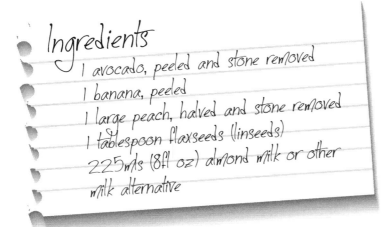

Ingredients
- 1 avocado, peeled and stone removed
- 1 banana, peeled
- 1 large peach, halved and stone removed
- 1 tablespoon flaxseeds (linseeds)
- 225mls (8fl oz) almond milk or other milk alternative

SERVES
1

Method

Place all of the ingredients into a blender and process until smooth. Serve and drink straight away.

Fresh Detox Smoothie

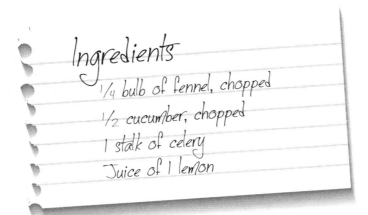

Ingredients
- 1/4 bulb of fennel, chopped
- 1/2 cucumber, chopped
- 1 stalk of celery
- Juice of 1 lemon

SERVES
1

Method

Place the all of the ingredients into a food processor or smoothie maker and pour in just enough water to cover the ingredients. Blitz until smooth.

Ginger & Avocado Cream Smoothie

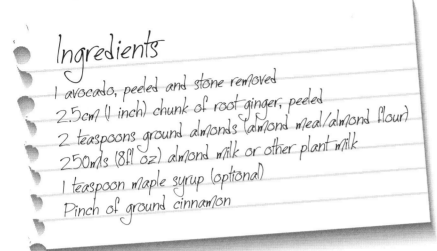

Ingredients

1 avocado, peeled and stone removed
2.5cm (1 inch) chunk of root ginger, peeled
2 teaspoons ground almonds (almond meal/almond flour)
250mls (8fl oz) almond milk or other plant milk
1 teaspoon maple syrup (optional)
Pinch of ground cinnamon

SERVES
1

Method

Place all of the ingredients into a food processor and blitz until smooth and creamy. Serve

Peanut Butter & Banana Smoothie

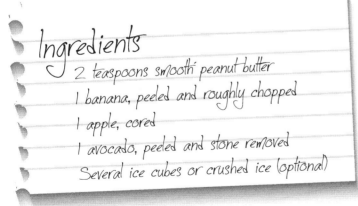

Ingredients

2 teaspoons smooth peanut butter
1 banana, peeled and roughly chopped
1 apple, cored
1 avocado, peeled and stone removed
Several ice cubes or crushed ice (optional)

SERVES
1

Method

Place all of the ingredients into a blender and blitz until smooth. If your blender doesn't tolerate ice you can just add a few cubes for serving.

Pink Grapefruit & Raspberry Blend

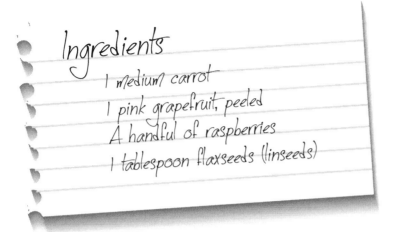

Ingredients

1 medium carrot
1 pink grapefruit, peeled
A handful of raspberries
1 tablespoon flaxseeds (linseeds)

SERVES 1

Method

Place all of the ingredients into a blender with enough water to cover them. Blitz until smooth. Enjoy.

Sweet Green Juice

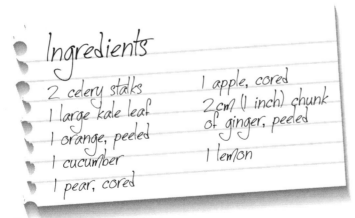

Ingredients

2 celery stalks
1 large kale leaf
1 orange, peeled
1 cucumber
1 pear, cored

1 apple, cored
2cm (1 inch) chunk of ginger, peeled
1 lemon

SERVES 1

Method

Process all of the ingredients through a juicer and pour the juice into a glass. Add a few ice cubes and drink straight away.

Lemon & Coconut Salad Smoothie

Ingredients

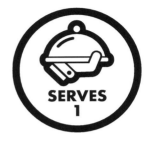

SERVES 1

1 large handful of lettuce leaves

1 apple, cored

1/2 cucumber

Juice of 1/2 lemon

250mls (8fl oz) coconut water (unsweetened)

Method

Place all of the ingredients into a blender and blitz until smooth. Serve straight away.

Berry Cocktail

Ingredients

SERVES 1

50g (2oz) blueberries

50g (2oz) strawberries, stalk removed

50g (2oz) raspberries

1 pear, cored

1 teaspoon of maca powder

A handful of spinach leaves

Method

Place the ingredients into a blender and add just enough water to cover the ingredients. Process until smooth.

Strawberry & Mint Smoothie

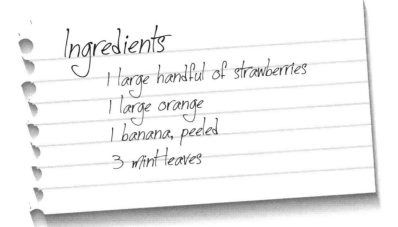

Ingredients

1 large handful of strawberries
1 large orange
1 banana, peeled
3 mint leaves

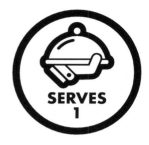

SERVES
1

Method

Place all of the ingredients into a food processor and add just enough water to cover them and process until smooth.

Fresh Ginger, Carrot and Avocado Smoothie

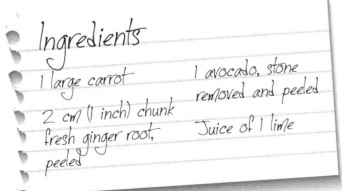

Ingredients

1 large carrot

2 cm (1 inch) chunk fresh ginger root, peeled

1 avocado, stone removed and peeled

Juice of 1 lime

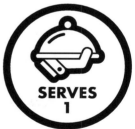

SERVES
1

Method

Place all the ingredients into a blender and blitz until smooth. Serve and enjoy.

Blueberry Overnight Oats

Ingredients

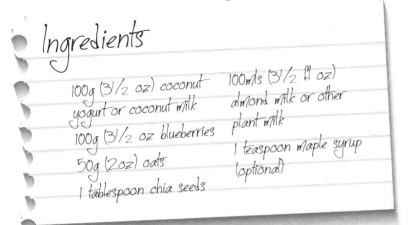

100g (3½ oz) coconut yogurt or coconut milk

100g (3½ oz) blueberries

50g (2oz) oats

1 tablespoon chia seeds

100mls (3½ fl oz) almond milk or other plant milk

1 teaspoon maple syrup (optional)

SERVES 1

Method

Place the oats in a glass jar or serving bowl. Add the coconut yogurt or coconut milk on top. Add the blueberries and pour the milk over the top. Cover and keep it in the fridge until ready to eat. You have a quick and healthy breakfast ready prepared.

Raspberry Chia Jam

Ingredients

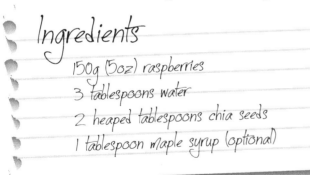

150g (5oz) raspberries

3 tablespoons water

2 heaped tablespoons chia seeds

1 tablespoon maple syrup (optional)

SERVES 1

Method

Place all of the ingredients in a saucepan and bring it to a simmer, stirring constantly. Mash the fruit to a pulp and cook for around 3 minutes, until the fruit is softened and the mixture has thickened. Allow it to cool and transfer it to a glass jar. Store refrigerated until ready to use. Serve with toast or pancakes.

Chickpea Pancakes

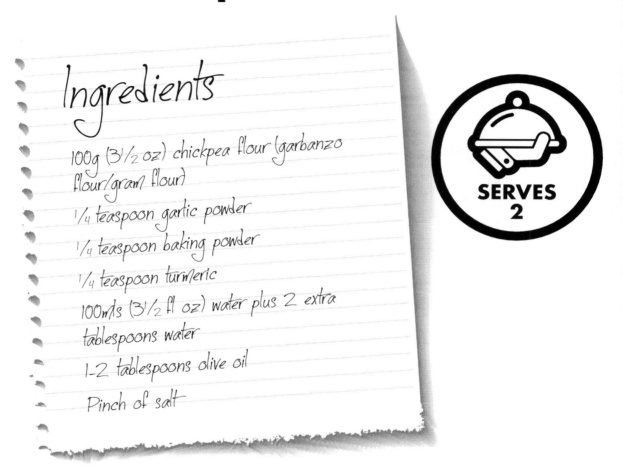

Ingredients

100g (3½ oz) chickpea flour (garbanzo flour/gram flour)

¼ teaspoon garlic powder

¼ teaspoon baking powder

¼ teaspoon turmeric

100mls (3½ fl oz) water plus 2 extra tablespoons water

1-2 tablespoons olive oil

Pinch of salt

SERVES 2

Method

In a bowl, mix together the chickpea flour (garbanzo flour/gram flour) garlic powder, baking powder, salt and turmeric. Slowly whisk in the water until you have a smooth batter. Heat the olive oil in a small frying pan. Pour half of the mixture into the pan and cook until golden then flip it over and cook on the other side. You can serve the pancakes with a wide variety of fillings like avocado, tahini, tomatoes, mushrooms, relish, fresh herbs, hummus, spinach, peppers, onions, cucumber, olives and legumes.

French Toast With Blueberries & Maple Syrup

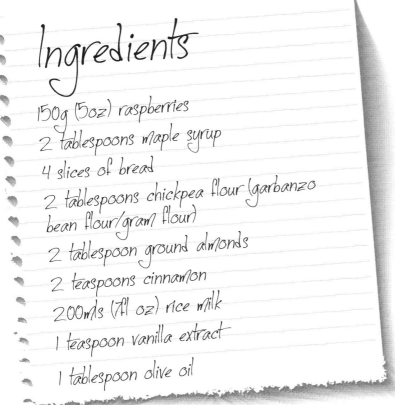

Ingredients

150g (5oz) raspberries

2 tablespoons maple syrup

4 slices of bread

2 tablespoons chickpea flour (garbanzo bean flour/gram flour)

2 tablespoon ground almonds

2 teaspoons cinnamon

200mls (7fl oz) rice milk

1 teaspoon vanilla extract

1 tablespoon olive oil

SERVES
4

Method

Place the flour, almonds, cinnamon, rice milk and vanilla in a bowl and whisk them together. Heat the olive oil in a frying pan. Dip the bread in the flour mixture, coating it well. Place the bread into the frying pan and cook until slightly golden then turn it over to cook on the other side. Serve with a drizzle of maple syrup and a scattering of blueberries. Enjoy it while it's hot.

Coconut Yogurt Almond Crunch

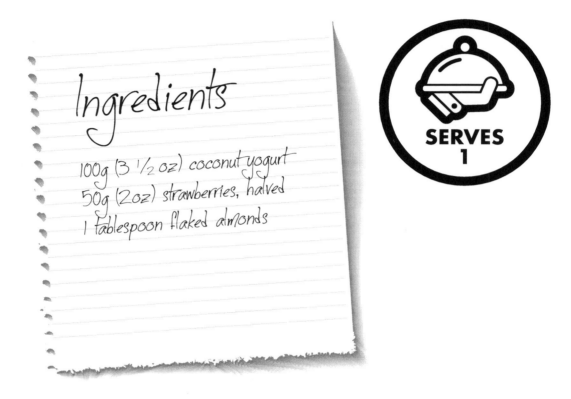

SERVES 1

Ingredients

100g (3 ½ oz) coconut yogurt
50g (2oz) strawberries, halved
1 tablespoon flaked almonds

Method

Mash together half of the strawberries with the coconut yogurt. Spoon half of the yogurt into a glass and add a layer of strawberries and almonds then add another layer of yogurt. Scatter some strawberries and almonds on top. Serve and eat straight away.

Quinoa & Raspberry Porridge

SERVES 1

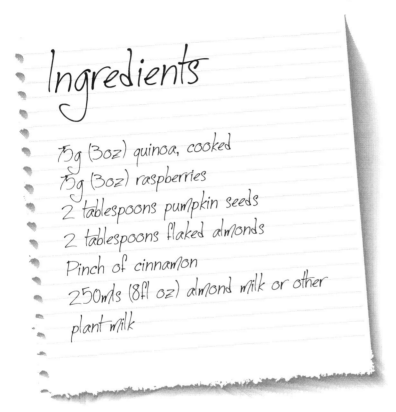

Ingredients

75g (3oz) quinoa, cooked

75g (3oz) raspberries

2 tablespoons pumpkin seeds

2 tablespoons flaked almonds

Pinch of cinnamon

250mls (8fl oz) almond milk or other

plant milk

Method

Pour the almond milk into a saucepan and add the quinoa. Bring it to the boil and cook for 5 minutes. Sprinkle in the cinnamon. Serve it into a bowl and scatter the pumpkin seeds and almonds on top, followed by the raspberries. Eat straight away.

Cinnamon & Pear Porridge

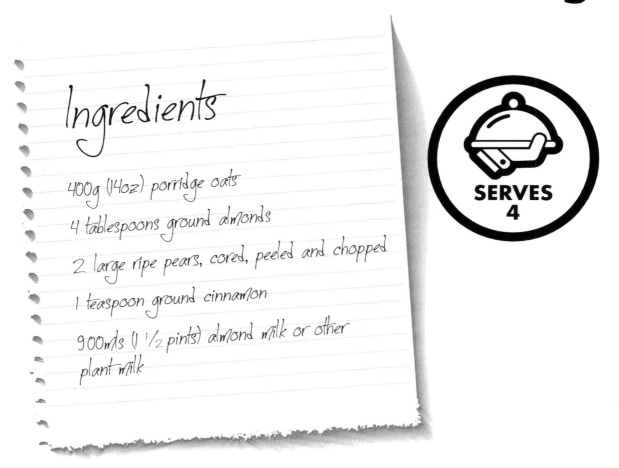

Ingredients

400g (14oz) porridge oats

4 tablespoons ground almonds

2 large ripe pears, cored, peeled and chopped

1 teaspoon ground cinnamon

900mls (1 ½ pints) almond milk or other plant milk

SERVES 4

Method

In a saucepan, cook all of the ingredients, apart from ground almonds, for 5 minutes or until it thickens. Serve topped with a sprinkling of ground almonds.

LUNCH

Miso Broth

Ingredients

225g (8oz) pak choi (bok choy), chopped
200g (7oz) tofu, cubed
10 spring onions (scallions), finely chopped
2 star anise
3 tablespoons red miso
1 tablespoon fresh coriander (cilantro), freshly chopped
1 small red chilli pepper
1/2 teaspoon ground ginger
1200mls (2 pints) vegetable stock (broth)
2 tablespoons tamari sauce

SERVES 4

Method

Place the pak choi (bok choy) into a saucepan with the ginger, star anise, coriander (cilantro), chilli and vegetable stock (broth). Bring it to the boil, reduce the heat and simmer for 5 minute. Add the spring onions (scallions), tamari sauce and tofu. Cook for 3 minutes. In a small bowl, blend the red miso with 3 tablespoons of the soup broth then stir it into the soup. Sprinkle in the coriander (cilantro) and serve.

Quick Red Pepper (Bell Pepper) & Basil Soup

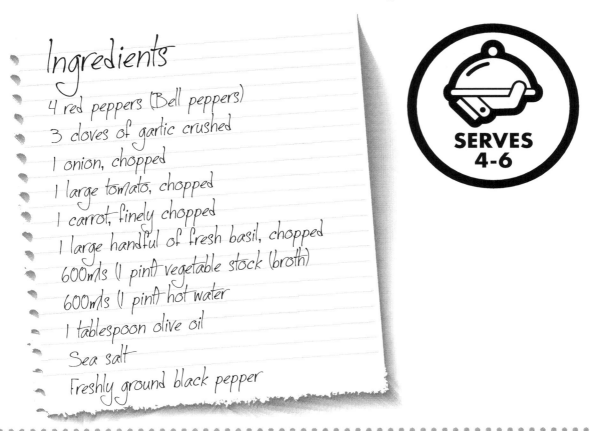

Ingredients

4 red peppers (Bell peppers)
3 cloves of garlic crushed
1 onion, chopped
1 large tomato, chopped
1 carrot, finely chopped
1 large handful of fresh basil, chopped
600mls (1 pint) vegetable stock (broth)
600mls (1 pint) hot water
1 tablespoon olive oil
Sea salt
Freshly ground black pepper

SERVES
4-6

Method

Heat the oil in a saucepan. Add the onion, carrot and garlic and cook for 3 minutes.
Add in the tomato and red peppers (bell peppers), hot water and stock and cook for
10 minutes. Add in the fresh basil. Using a hand blender or food processor, blitz the soup
until smooth. Season with salt and pepper and serve. Serve and enjoy.

Fast & Tasty Tomato Soup

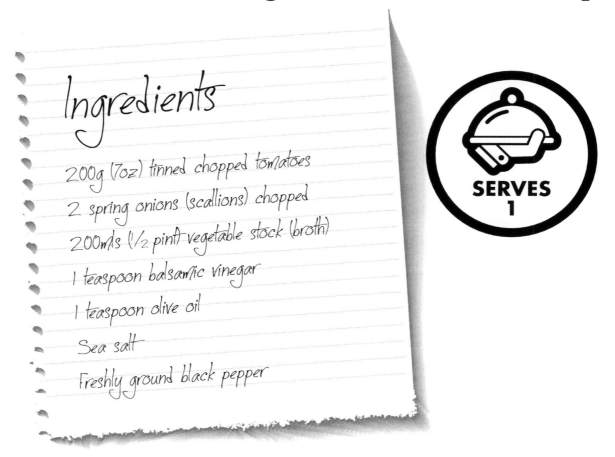

Ingredients

200g (7oz) tinned chopped tomatoes

2 spring onions (scallions) chopped

200mls (½ pint) vegetable stock (broth)

1 teaspoon balsamic vinegar

1 teaspoon olive oil

Sea salt

Freshly ground black pepper

SERVES 1

Method

Heat the oil in a saucepan, add the spring onions (scallions) and cook for 2 minutes. Add in the tomatoes and stock (broth) and bring it to the boil. Add in a teaspoon of balsamic vinegar. Reduce the heat and simmer for 5 minutes until heated through. Using a food processor and or hand blender blitz until smooth. Season with salt and pepper. Enjoy.

Cauliflower & Walnut Soup

Ingredients

450g (1lb) cauliflower, finely chopped

1 onion, chopped

2 tablespoons chopped walnuts

600mls (1½ pints) hot water

125mls (4fl oz) almond milk or other plant milk

1 tablespoon olive oil

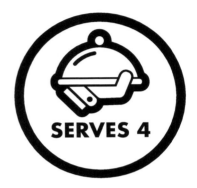

SERVES 4

Method

Heat the oil in a saucepan, add the cauliflower and onion and cook for 2 minutes, stirring continuously. Pour in the hot water, bring to the boil and cook for 10 minutes. Stir in the almond milk. Using a food processor or hand blender, blitz the soup until smooth and creamy. Serve with a sprinkling of walnuts and enjoy.

Asparagus Soup

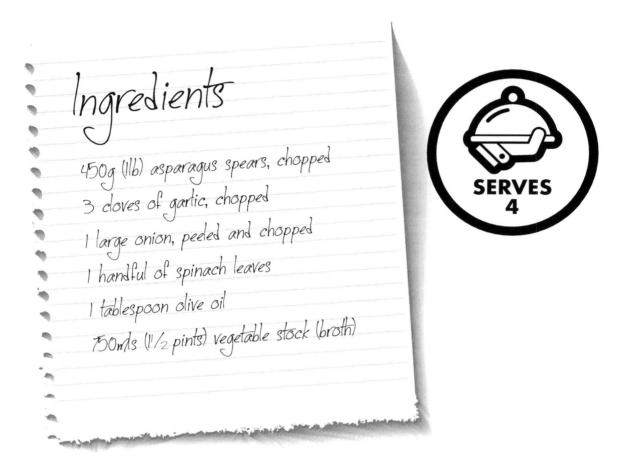

Ingredients

450g (1lb) asparagus spears, chopped

3 cloves of garlic, chopped

1 large onion, peeled and chopped

1 handful of spinach leaves

1 tablespoon olive oil

750mls (1½ pints) vegetable stock (broth)

**SERVES
4**

Method

Heat the oil in a saucepan, add the onion, garlic and asparagus and cook for 4 minutes. Add in the spinach and vegetable stock (broth) and cook for 5 minutes. Using a hand blender or food processor blitz the soup until smooth. Serve into bowls.

Gazpacho

Ingredients

- 10 tomatoes, de-seeded and chopped
- 5 cloves of garlic, chopped
- 2 red peppers (bell peppers), de-seeded and chopped
- 2 medium cucumbers, peeled and chopped
- 1 teaspoon chilli flakes
- 4 tablespoons apple cider vinegar
- 4 teaspoons olive oil
- Sea salt
- Freshly ground black pepper

SERVES 4

Method

Place all of the ingredients into a food processor or blender and blitz until smooth. If the soup is too thick, just add a little extra oil or vinegar. Eat straight away or chill in the fridge before serving.

Red Pepper & Chickpea Soup

SERVES 4

Ingredients

200g (6oz) tinned chickpeas (garbanzo beans), drained

3 red peppers (bell pepper), de-seeded and chopped

2 teaspoons ground coriander (cilantro)

1 onion, peeled and chopped

1 handful of fresh parsley, chopped

1½ litres (2½ pints) vegetable stock (broth)

1 tablespoon olive oil

Method

Heat the oil in a large saucepan, add the onion and cook for 2 minutes. Add in the red peppers (bell pepper), ground coriander (cilantro) and stock (broth). Bring it to the boil, reduce the heat and simmer until the vegetables have softened. Using a hand blender or food processor and blitz until smooth. Return it to the saucepan, add the parsley and chickpeas (garbanzo beans) and warm them. Serve and enjoy.

Mediterranean Tomato & Lentil Soup

Ingredients

SERVES 4

400g (14oz) tin of chopped tomatoes
350g (12oz) tinned cooked lentils (drained)
1 large onion, peeled and chopped
1 teaspoon tomato purée (paste)
1 teaspoon dried mixed herbs
1 tablespoon olive oil
900mls (1½ pints) hot vegetable stock (broth)
A large handful of fresh basil leaves, chopped

Method

Heat the oil in a frying pan, add the onion and cook for 4 minutes. Add in the vegetable stock (broth), tomatoes, lentils and dried mixed herbs and bring it to the boil. Simmer for around 5 minutes. Stir in the basil. Use a food processor or hand blender and process until smooth. Serve and enjoy.

Buddha Bowls

Ingredients

100g (3½ oz) cooked beans or lentils
75g (3oz) cooked (preferably roasted) chopped sweet potatoes
50g (2oz) red cabbage, finely chopped
1 packet of cooked wholegrain rice or quinoa
1 avocado, stone removed, peeled and sliced
1 tablespoon cashew nuts
1 teaspoon sesame seeds
½ teaspoon paprika
½ teaspoon chilli flakes
1 small handful of fresh coriander (cilantro)

FOR THE DRESSING:

1 tablespoon tahini
1 teaspoon lemon juice
1 tablespoon water
Pinch of cayenne pepper
Pinch of sea salt

Method

Put the tahini, lemon juice, water, cayenne pepper and salt into a bowl and mix well. Add a little water or extra lemon juice if it seems too thick. Assemble your Buddha bowl starting at the bottom with the rice or quinoa. Add the sweet potatoes, avocado, cabbage, beans/lentils, nuts and seeds in individual piles on top. Sprinkle over the paprika, chilli and coriander (cilantro). Drizzle the dressing over the ingredients. Eat straight away.

The key to fast and tasty Buddha bowls is leftovers. Cook extra potatoes, vegetables and bean dishes to save time and energy preparing them from scratch, that way you can assemble a Buddha bowl straight from ingredients you already have in the fridge. The varieties you can make are endless. This recipe is for a basic Buddha bowl but you can include almost anything you like. You can use leftover roast vegetables, falafels, tofu, guacamole, couscous, hummus, sliced apple, grated carrots, celery, tomatoes, cauliflower, broccoli, spinach, sweetcorn and add a handful of nuts, seeds and fresh herbs. Add plenty of colours for vibrancy and great nutrition. Dressings will add even more variety and there are more recipes for these at the back.

Creamy Courgette 'Spaghetti' & Pine Nuts

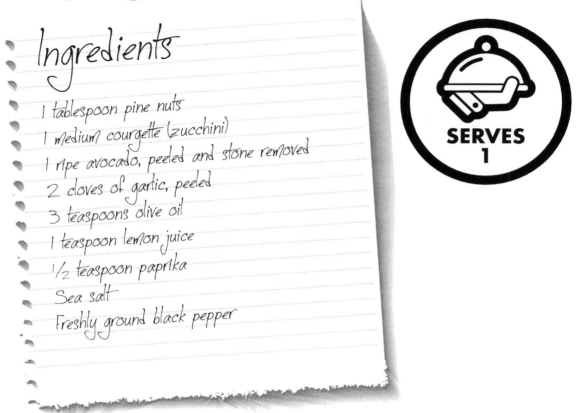

Ingredients

1 tablespoon pine nuts

1 medium courgette (zucchini)

1 ripe avocado, peeled and stone removed

2 cloves of garlic, peeled

3 teaspoons olive oil

1 teaspoon lemon juice

½ teaspoon paprika

Sea salt

Freshly ground black pepper

SERVES 1

Method

Use a spiraliser or if you don't have one, use a vegetable peeler and cut the courgette (zucchini) into thin strips. Heat 2 teaspoons of oil in a frying pan, add the courgette (zucchini) and cook for 4-5 minutes or until it has softened. In the meantime, place the avocado paprika, garlic, lemon juice and a teaspoon of olive oil into a blender and blitz the mixture until smooth. Add the avocado mixture to the pan with the courgette (zucchini) and stir it well until warmed through. Season with salt and pepper. Serve and sprinkle with pine nuts.

Lemon & Pine Nut Asparagus

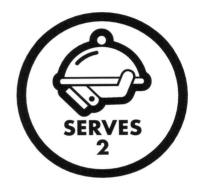

SERVES 2

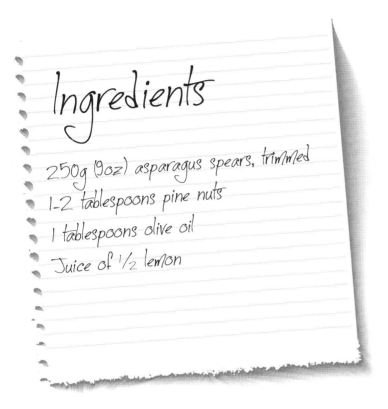

Ingredients

250g (9oz) asparagus spears, trimmed

1-2 tablespoons pine nuts

1 tablespoons olive oil

Juice of ½ lemon

Method

Coat a griddle pan or frying pan with olive oil. Lay out the asparagus spears on it and squeeze the lemon juice on top. Cook for 6 minutes, turning occasionally. Scatter the pine nuts into the pan and warm them slightly. Serve and eat straight away.

Bean & Chilli Pineapple Salad

Ingredients

- 400g (14oz) cannellini beans (or other bean if preferred)
- 200g (7oz) pineapple, chopped
- 2 large handfuls of spinach leaves
- 1 small onion, finely chopped
- 2.5cm (1inch) chunk of fresh ginger, peel and finely chopped
- ½ teaspoon garam masala
- ½ teaspoon ground cumin
- ¼ teaspoon turmeric
- A handful of coriander (cilantro), finely chopped
- 1 tablespoon olive oil

SERVES 2

Method

Place the cumin, garam masala, turmeric and olive oil into a bowl and mix well. Place all the remaining ingredients into a bowl and pour the dressing over them. Stir well and serve.

Mexican Rice & Bean Salad

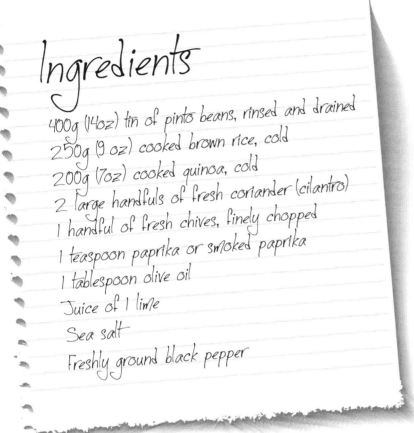

Ingredients

400g (14oz) tin of pinto beans, rinsed and drained
250g (9 oz) cooked brown rice, cold
200g (7oz) cooked quinoa, cold
2 large handfuls of fresh coriander (cilantro)
1 handful of fresh chives, finely chopped
1 teaspoon paprika or smoked paprika
1 tablespoon olive oil
Juice of 1 lime
Sea salt
Freshly ground black pepper

SERVES
2

Method

Place the beans, rice, quinoa, coriander (cilantro), chives, paprika, olive oil and lime juice into a bowl and mix well. Season with salt and pepper. Chill before serving.

Beetroot & Lentil Salad

Ingredients

- 200g (7oz) tinned cooked Puy lentils
- 100g (3½ oz) cooked beetroot, sliced
- 2 tomatoes, deseeded and chopped
- 4 spring onions (scallions), finely chopped
- 1 tablespoon olive oil
- 1 small handful of parsley, chopped
- 1 small handful of fresh basil leaves, chopped
- 1 large handful of washed spinach leaves
- 2 cloves of garlic, finely chopped
- Juice and rind of 1 lime
- Sea salt
- Freshly ground black pepper

SERVES 1

Method

Heat the olive oil in a saucepan, add the garlic and spring onions (scallions) and cook for 1 minute. Add the tomatoes, lentils, lime juice and rind. Cook for 2 minutes. Sprinkle in the herbs and stir. Scatter the spinach leaves and beetroot and serve the lentils on top. Season with salt and pepper.

Cannellini Beans & Spinach

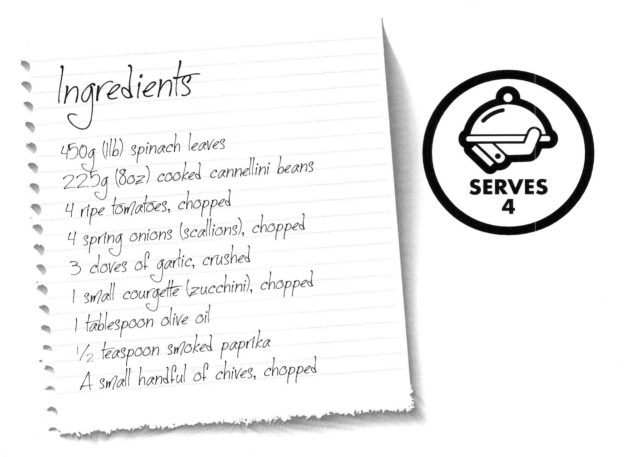

Ingredients

450g (1lb) spinach leaves
225g (8oz) cooked cannellini beans
4 ripe tomatoes, chopped
4 spring onions (scallions), chopped
3 cloves of garlic, crushed
1 small courgette (zucchini), chopped
1 tablespoon olive oil
1/2 teaspoon smoked paprika
A small handful of chives, chopped

SERVES
4

Method

Heat the olive oil in a frying pan and add the garlic, courgette (zucchini) and tomatoes and cook until softened. Add in the spinach, spring onions (scallions) and cannellini beans, chives and smoked paprika and cook until the spinach wilts. Serve with a sprinkling of chives.

Sweetcorn & Bean Salad

Ingredients

225g (8oz) tin of sweetcorn, drained

400g (14oz) tin of pinto beans, drained and rinsed

400g (14oz) tin of blackbeans, drained and rinsed

8 spring onions (scallions), chopped

4 tomatoes, chopped

1 handful of fresh coriander (cilantro) chopped

1 handful of fresh chives, chopped

1 clove of garlic, finely chopped

1 teaspoon sea salt

1 avocado, stone removed, peeled and diced

1 red pepper (bell pepper), chopped

1 green pepper (bell pepper), chopped

1 teaspoon paprika powder

1/2 teaspoon chilli powder (optional)

6 tablespoons olive oil

Juice of 1 lemon

SERVES 4

Method

Place the lemon juice, olive oil, paprika powder, garlic, salt and chilli in a bowl and mix well. In a large serving bowl, combine the beans, sweetcorn, avocado, tomatoes, peppers (bell peppers), spring onions (scallions), chives and coriander (cilantro). Pour the oil mixture over the salad ingredients and mix well before serving

Grapefruit & Pine Nut Salad

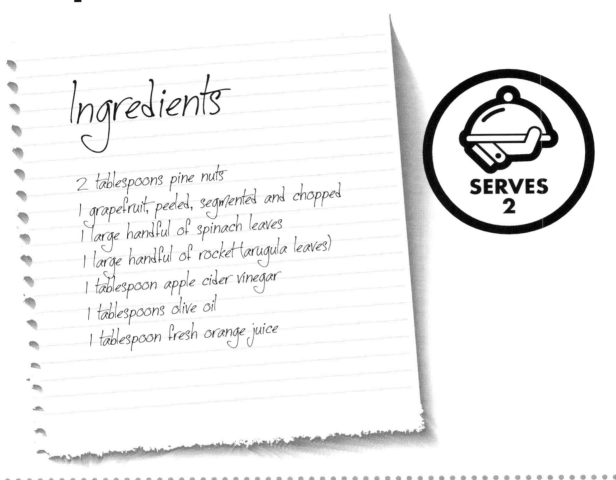

Ingredients

2 tablespoons pine nuts
1 grapefruit, peeled, segmented and chopped
1 large handful of spinach leaves
1 large handful of rocket (arugula leaves)
1 tablespoon apple cider vinegar
1 tablespoons olive oil
1 tablespoon fresh orange juice

SERVES 2

Method

Pour the oil, vinegar and juice into a bowl and toss the grapefruit, spinach and rocket (arugula) leaves in the mixture. Serve onto plates and sprinkle some pine nuts on top. Enjoy.

Linguine

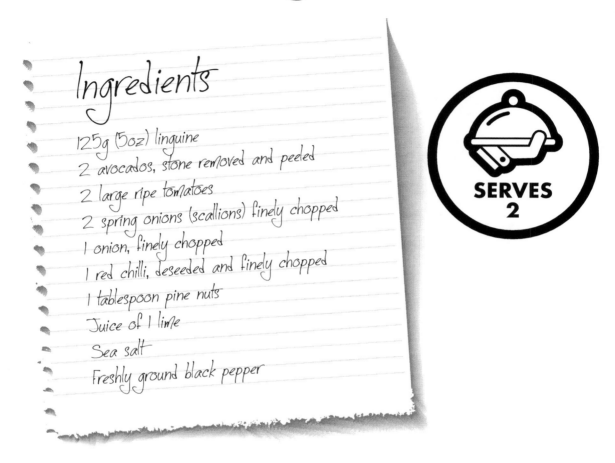

Ingredients

125g (5oz) linguine
2 avocados, stone removed and peeled
2 large ripe tomatoes
2 spring onions (scallions) finely chopped
1 onion, finely chopped
1 red chilli, deseeded and finely chopped
1 tablespoon pine nuts
Juice of 1 lime
Sea salt
Freshly ground black pepper

SERVES 2

Method

Place the pasta in hot water and cook according to the instructions. In the meantime put the tomatoes, avocados, onion, lime, basil and chilli into a large bowl. When the pasta has cooked, drain it and add it to the bowl. Toss the pasta in the vegetable mixture. Season with salt and pepper and sprinkle on the pine nuts. Can be eaten hot or cold.

Melted Cheesy Courgettes

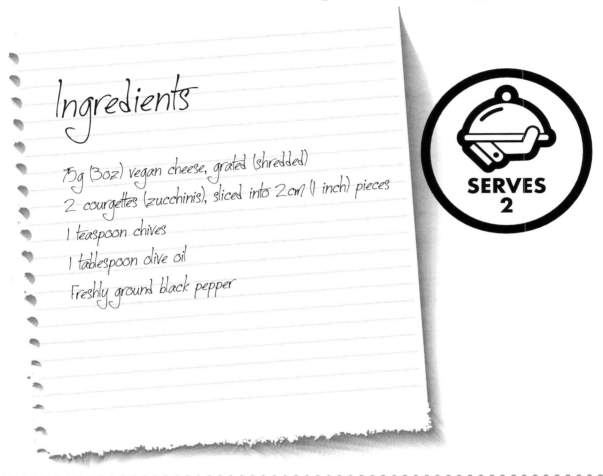

Ingredients

75g (3oz) vegan cheese, grated (shredded)

2 courgettes (zucchinis), sliced into 2cm (1 inch) pieces

1 teaspoon chives

1 tablespoon olive oil

Freshly ground black pepper

SERVES 2

Method

Heat the oil in a frying pan. Add the courgette (zucchini) and cook for around 2 minutes on each side. Lay the courgette (zucchini) slices on a baking sheet and sprinkle over the vegan cheese and chives. Place under a hot grill (broiler) for 3-4 minutes until the cheese melts. Season with black pepper. Serve and eat straight away.

Cauliflower 'Steak' Burgers

SERVES 2

Ingredients

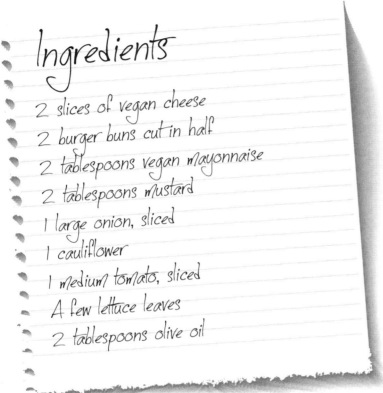

2 slices of vegan cheese

2 burger buns cut in half

2 tablespoons vegan mayonnaise

2 tablespoons mustard

1 large onion, sliced

1 cauliflower

1 medium tomato, sliced

A few lettuce leaves

2 tablespoons olive oil

Method

Remove any leaves from the cauliflower. With the stalk facing down onto a chopping board, cut 2 x 2cm (1 inch) thick slices from the middle of the cauliflower so you have ample stalk holding the florets together. Save the remaining cauliflower to use at another time.

Heat the olive oil in a frying pan, add the cauliflower slices and cook on a high heat until they are golden, then turn them over and cook on the other side. In the meantime, add the onion to one side of the frying pan and cook them until soft. Put a little lettuce in each burger bun and add some vegan mayo and a slice of tomato. Place the cauliflower (burger) inside the bun, add some mustard and onion. Add a slice of cheese on top and the other half of the bun. Enjoy straight away.

Cream 'Cheese' & Chives

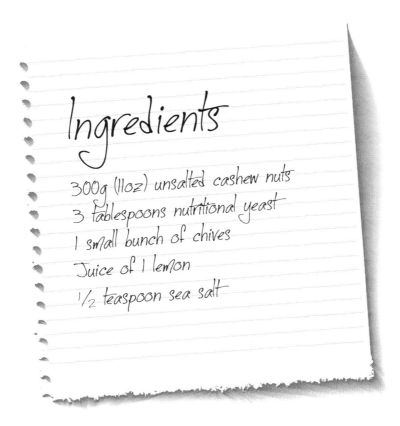

Ingredients

300g (11oz) unsalted cashew nuts
3 tablespoons nutritional yeast
1 small bunch of chives
Juice of 1 lemon
½ teaspoon sea salt

Method

A little preparation is required to make this but it's otherwise very quick and simple to make. Simply put the cashews in a bowl of water, cover it and soak them overnight.

Drain the water off the cashews and place them in a food processor along with the yeast and lemon juice and blend them until they are completely smooth. Spoon the 'cheese' into a bowl and add in the chopped chives. Keep refrigerated until ready to eat. Spread it on fresh bread and crackers or use it as a dip with crudités.

DINNER

Vegan Meatballs & Tomato Sauce

Ingredients

400g (14oz) tin of chickpeas

75g (3oz) tin of peas

2 cloves of garlic, chopped
or ready-chopped garlic

1 jar of ready-made tomato
and basil sauce

1 red onion, peeled and
chopped

1 red pepper
(bell pepper), deseeded
and roughly chopped

1 handful of spinach

1 teaspoon paprika

1 teaspoon onion powder

2 tablespoons gram flour
(chickpea/garbanzo flour)

2 tablespoons olive oil

Sunflower oil for cooking

Extra gram flour for rolling

**SERVES
2**

Method

Heat the olive oil in a frying pan and add the onion, pepper and garlic and cook for 3 minutes.
Transfer them to a food processor and add in the chickpeas (garbanzo beans), peas, spinach,
paprika, onion powder, gram flour (chickpea flour/garbanzo bean flour) and sunflower oil.
The mixture should be soft and slightly sticky, ready to roll into balls. If you need extra liquid try
adding a little extra oil or a tablespoon or two of water. Take a spoonful of the mixture and roll
it into a ball then coat it in a little gram flour. Cook the balls in hot oil in the frying pan until
golden. Heat the tomato sauce and serve the 'meatballs' with the sauce and spaghetti or pasta.

Quick Thai Vegetable Curry

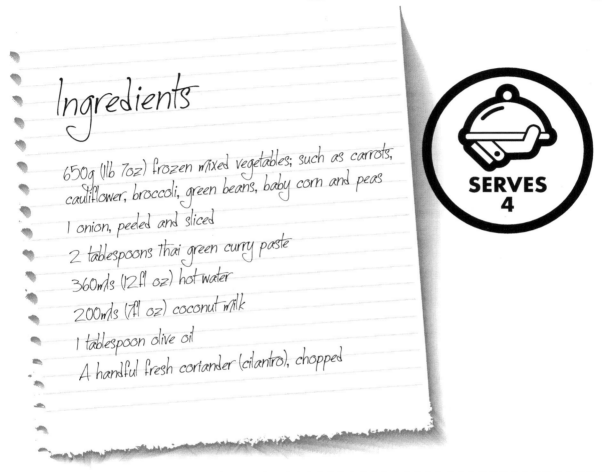

Ingredients

650g (1lb 7oz) frozen mixed vegetables; such as carrots, cauliflower, broccoli, green beans, baby corn and peas

1 onion, peeled and sliced

2 tablespoons thai green curry paste

360mls (12fl oz) hot water

200mls (7fl oz) coconut milk

1 tablespoon olive oil

A handful fresh coriander (cilantro), chopped

SERVES 4

Method

Heat the oil in a large saucepan. Add the onion and cook for 2 minutes. Add the vegetables and add the curry paste, coconut milk and the hot water. Cover and cook until the vegetables have softened. Stir in the coriander (cilantro). Serve with rice.

Pesto Pepper & Tofu Kebabs

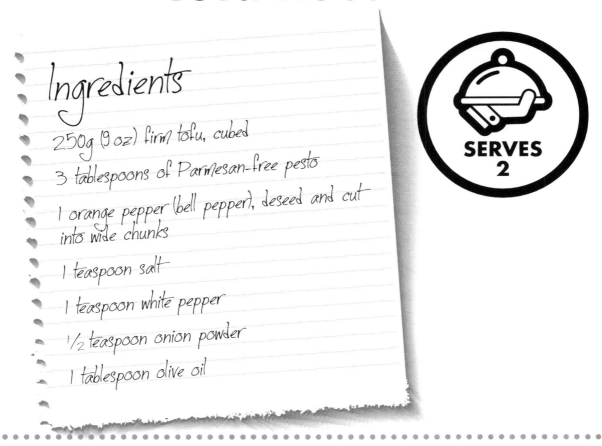

SERVES
2

Ingredients

250g (9 oz) firm tofu, cubed

3 tablespoons of Parmesan-free pesto

1 orange pepper (bell pepper), deseed and cut into wide chunks

1 teaspoon salt

1 teaspoon white pepper

1/2 teaspoon onion powder

1 tablespoon olive oil

Method

Place the orange pepper (bell pepper), pesto, salt, pepper, onion powder and olive oil into a bowl and mix well. Add the tofu and gently coat it in the mixture. Thread the tofu and vegetables alternately onto metal skewers (if using bamboo skewers you will need to soak them in water first). Place the skewers under a hot preheated grill (broiler) and cook them for around 3 minutes on each side, turning them occasionally. Alternatively they can be cooked on a barbeque. Serve with rice, quinoa or salad.

Tacos & Avocado Dressing

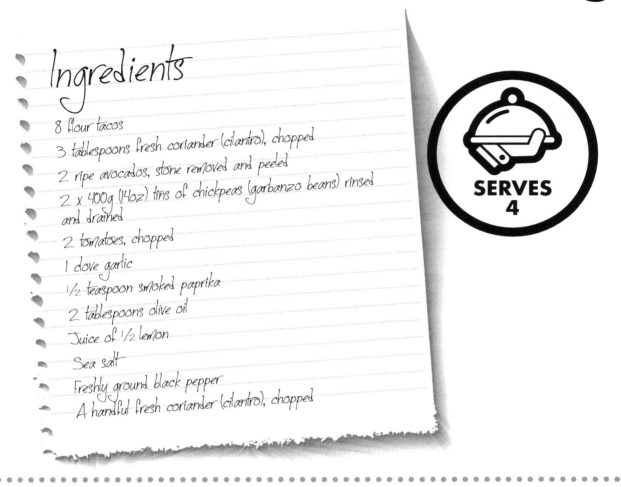

Ingredients

- 8 flour tacos
- 3 tablespoons fresh coriander (cilantro), chopped
- 2 ripe avocados, stone removed and peeled
- 2 x 400g (14oz) tins of chickpeas (garbanzo beans) rinsed and drained
- 2 tomatoes, chopped
- 1 clove garlic
- 1/2 teaspoon smoked paprika
- 2 tablespoons olive oil
- Juice of 1/2 lemon
- Sea salt
- Freshly ground black pepper
- A handful fresh coriander (cilantro), chopped

SERVES 4

Method

Place the chickpeas (garbanzo beans) into a large bowl and mash them. Add in the coriander (cilantro), tomatoes, smoked paprika and garlic and mix well. Season with salt and pepper. Place the avocado flesh into a food processor along with the lemon juice, garlic and olive oil and process until creamy. Spoon the chickpea mixture into the tacos and add a spoonful of the avocado mixture into each one. You can add extra filling like lettuce, onion, sweetcorn, cucumber and tahini.

Smoked Mushroom & Vegetable Skewers

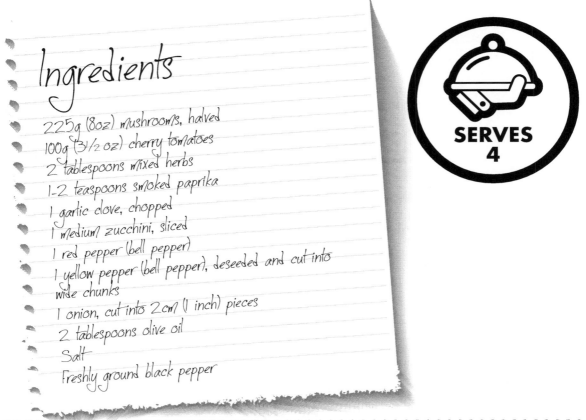

SERVES 4

Ingredients

225g (8oz) mushrooms, halved
100g (3½ oz) cherry tomatoes
2 tablespoons mixed herbs
1-2 teaspoons smoked paprika
1 garlic clove, chopped
1 medium zucchini, sliced
1 red pepper (bell pepper)
1 yellow pepper (bell pepper), deseeded and cut into wide chunks
1 onion, cut into 2cm (1 inch) pieces
2 tablespoons olive oil
Salt
Freshly ground black pepper

Method

Place the oil, garlic, smoked paprika and herbs into a bowl and mix well. Add all the remaining ingredients into the bowl and coat them in the oil mixture. Season with salt and pepper. Thread the vegetables alternately onto metal skewers (if you use bamboo skewers you will need to soak them in water first). Place the skewers under a hot pre-heated grill (broiler) and cook for around 3-4 minutes on each side.

Speedy Bean Chilli

Ingredients

250g (9 oz) tinned of mixed beans, drained and rinsed

200mls (7fl oz) tomato passata or tinned chopped tomatoes

1 teaspoon Cajun seasoning

1 teaspoon ground cumin

1 teaspoon dried oregano

1/2 teaspoon paprika

1/2 teaspoon chili powder

Sea salt

Freshly ground black pepper

SERVES 2

Method

Place all of your ingredients into a saucepan, bring them to the boil and reduce the heat. Simmer for 10 minutes until the mixture is thoroughly warmed. Serve with rice and add a salsa and guacamole or salad.

Hearty Vegetable Stir-Fry

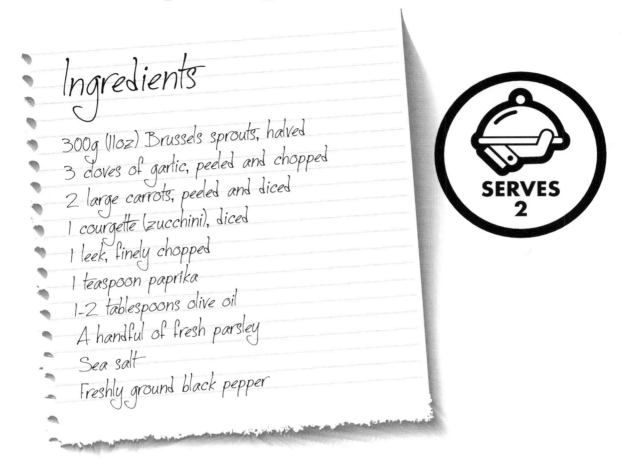

Ingredients

- 300g (11oz) Brussels sprouts, halved
- 3 cloves of garlic, peeled and chopped
- 2 large carrots, peeled and diced
- 1 courgette (zucchini), diced
- 1 leek, finely chopped
- 1 teaspoon paprika
- 1-2 tablespoons olive oil
- A handful of fresh parsley
- Sea salt
- Freshly ground black pepper

SERVES 2

Method

Heat the oil in a wok or frying pan. Add in the Brussels sprouts, courgette (zucchini), leek, carrots and garlic. Cook for around 5 minutes until the vegetables have softened. Sprinkle in the paprika and parsley. Season with salt and pepper before serving.

Spicy Quesadillas

Ingredients

200g (7oz) pinto beans, roughly mashed

75g (3oz) chickpeas (garbanzo beans), drained and mashed

4 spring onions (scallions), finely chopped

2 large wholemeal tortillas

1 large tomato, chopped

1 tablespoon almond butter

1 tablespoon tomato purée (paste)

1/2 teaspoon ground cumin

1/2 teaspoon dried oregano

1/2 teaspoon chilli powder (or more, if you like)

1/2 red pepper (bell pepper), finely chopped

1 tablespoon fresh coriander (cilantro), chopped

SERVES 2

Method

Spread each of the tortillas with some almond butter. Lay one tortilla flat in a dry frying pan. Scatter all of the remaining ingredients, apart from the coriander (cilantro) on top. Lay the other tortilla on top. Cook for 2-3 minutes, until warmed through. Serve with a sprinkling of coriander (cilantro). Eat straight away.

Falafels

Ingredients

- 400g (14oz) panko breadcrumbs
- 3 cloves of garlic, peeled
- 2 x 400g (14oz) tins of chickpeas (garbanzo beans)
- 2 red chillies, chopped
- 2 teaspoons ground cumin
- 2 teaspoons ground coriander
- 1/2 teaspoon baking powder
- 1/2 teaspoon turmeric
- 1 small onion, chopped
- 1 small handful of fresh coriander (cilantro) chopped
- 1 small handful of fresh flat leaf parsley
- Juice of 1 lime

SERVES 4

Method

Place all of the ingredients into a food processor and mix until smooth. Using clean hands, take a small amount of the mixture and roll it into a small bite-size ball. Repeat for all the remaining mixture. You can either deep fry the falafels if you like them really crispy or cook them in hot oil in a griddle pan. Serve hot or cold. They are so versatile and can be added to salads, served with dips or as a filling for sandwiches and pitta bread.

Ramon Noodles

Ingredients

450g (1lb) mushrooms, halved
200g (7oz) block of tofu
4 tablespoons red curry paste
2 spring onions (scallions)
1 red onion
1 tablespoon coconut oil (or olive oil)
1 pack of noodles
1 small bunch of fresh coriander (cilantro)

1 teaspoon ground ginger
½ teaspoon Tabasco sauce
1 teaspoon maple syrup
1.4 litres vegetable stock (broth)
400mls (14oz) tin coconut milk
75mls (3fl oz) soy sauce
Sprinkling of sesame seeds

SERVES 4

Method

Heat the olive oil in a large saucepan pan, add the onion, mushroom, soy sauce, Tabasco sauce, red curry paste and ginger and cook for 2 minutes. Add the stock (broth) and maple syrup and cook for 2 minutes. Pour in the coconut milk and bring it to a simmer. While it's cooking, cut the block of tofu into slices and place it under a hot grill (broiler) until crisp. Cook the noodles according to the instructions. Serve the noodles into bowls and divide the mushroom mixture between them. Add the tofu on top and sprinkle with sesame seeds, spring onions (scallions) and coriander (cilantro).

Sweet & Spicy Tofu

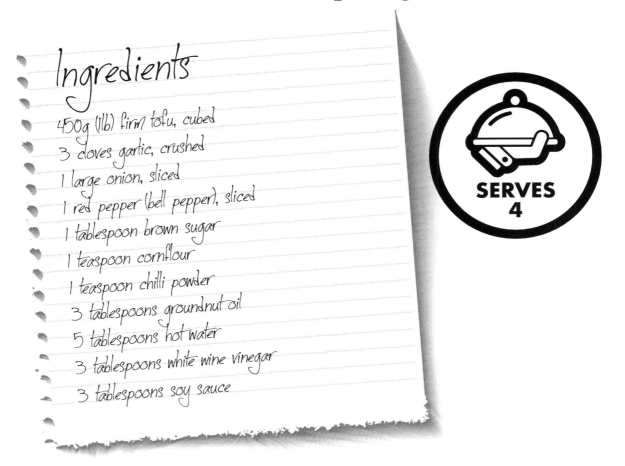

Ingredients

- 450g (1lb) firm tofu, cubed
- 3 cloves garlic, crushed
- 1 large onion, sliced
- 1 red pepper (bell pepper), sliced
- 1 tablespoon brown sugar
- 1 teaspoon cornflour
- 1 teaspoon chilli powder
- 3 tablespoons groundnut oil
- 5 tablespoons hot water
- 3 tablespoons white wine vinegar
- 3 tablespoons soy sauce

SERVES 4

Method

Heat the oil in a large frying pan or wok and brown it slightly. Add the onion, red pepper (bell pepper), garlic and chilli and cook for around 4 minutes or until slightly softened. In a bowl, mix together the soy sauce, hot water, vinegar, brown sugar and cornflour. Pour the mixture over the tofu and stir it well until it thickens slightly. Serve with rice.

Sweet Potato Noodles & Peanut Sauce

Ingredients

FOR THE PEANUT SAUCE:

50g (2oz) smooth peanut butter

2 tablespoons rice wine vinegar

2 tablespoons soy sauce

2 tablespoons toasted sesame oil

1 teaspoon ground ginger

1 garlic clove, chopped

120mls (4fl oz) warm water

FOR THE NOODLES:

2 spring onions (scallions), chopped

1 medium sweet potato, peeled and spiralised

1 large handful of spinach

1 tablespoon olive oil

SERVES 1

Method

Place all the ingredients for the satay sauce into a bowl and combine them thoroughly. Use a spiraliser to shred the sweet potato into 'noodles'. If you don't have a spiraliser, you can use a vegetable peeler to cut strips and then cut them lengthways. Heat the oil in a frying pan, add the sweet potato and cook for 5 minutes, stirring occasionally. Add in the spring onions (scallions) and spinach and cook until the spinach has wilted. Add the satay sauce and stir until the sauce is warmed through and has thickened. Serve and eat straight away.

Broccoli & Garlic Pasta

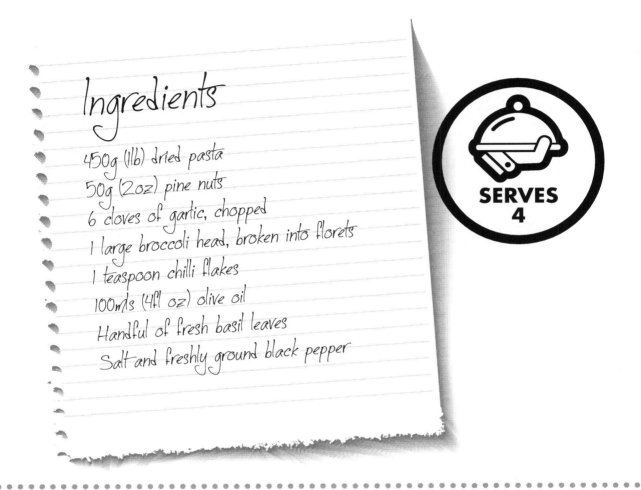

Ingredients

450g (1lb) dried pasta

50g (2oz) pine nuts

6 cloves of garlic, chopped

1 large broccoli head, broken into florets

1 teaspoon chilli flakes

100mls (4fl oz) olive oil

Handful of fresh basil leaves

Salt and freshly ground black pepper

SERVES 4

Method

Place the broccoli in a large saucepan of hot water and boil for 4 minutes or until tender. In the meantime, heat the olive oil in a large frying pan, add the garlic and chilli and cook for 2 minutes. Keep the boiling water and remove the broccoli using a slotted draining spoon and add it to the frying pan. Gently add the pasta to the boiling water and cook it according to the instructions. Add 100mls (3fl oz) hot water to the frying pan of broccoli and mash it along together with the chilli and garlic. Season with salt and pepper. Drain the pasta and transfer it to a large bowl. Spoon the broccoli over the top and mix in the basil leaves. Scatter the pine nuts over the top.

Mild Spiced Couscous

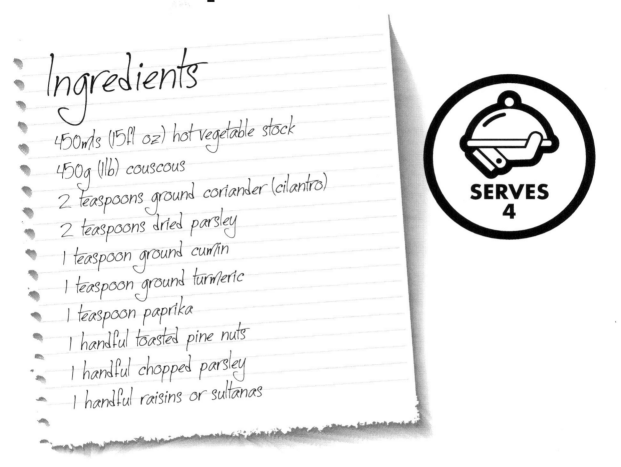

Ingredients

450mls (15fl oz) hot vegetable stock

450g (1lb) couscous

2 teaspoons ground coriander (cilantro)

2 teaspoons dried parsley

1 teaspoon ground cumin

1 teaspoon ground turmeric

1 teaspoon paprika

1 handful toasted pine nuts

1 handful chopped parsley

1 handful raisins or sultanas

SERVES 4

Method

Pour the vegetable stock over the couscous. Cover couscous and let rest for 10 minutes. Mix the spices and dried herbs together. Stir the spice mixture, pine nuts, chopped parsley and sultanas into the couscous. Mix everything together, ensuring the couscous is well flaked.

Wholegrain Rice Pilaf

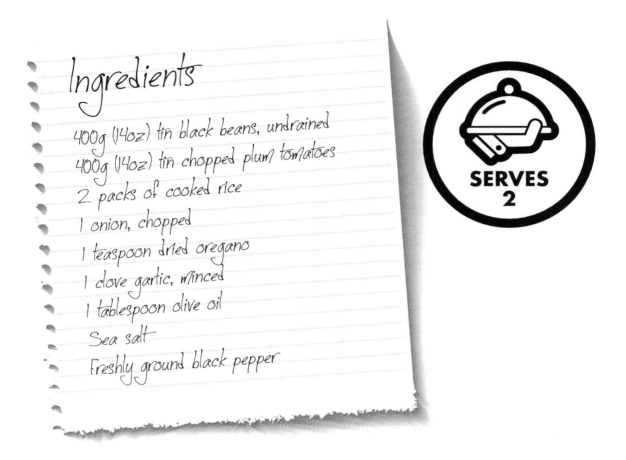

Ingredients

400g (14oz) tin black beans, undrained

400g (14oz) tin chopped plum tomatoes

2 packs of cooked rice

1 onion, chopped

1 teaspoon dried oregano

1 clove garlic, minced

1 tablespoon olive oil

Sea salt

Freshly ground black pepper

SERVES 2

Method

Heat the oil in a saucepan. Add the garlic and onion and cook until it softens. Add the beans, tomatoes, and oregano, bring it to the boil and add the rice. Simmer for 5 minutes. Season with salt and pepper and serve.

Tomato & Mushroom Spaghetti

Ingredients

400g (14oz) tinned tomatoes
300g (11oz) spaghetti
250g (9oz) mushrooms, sliced
3 cloves of garlic, chopped
1 stalk of celery, chopped
1 onion, peeled and chopped
1/2 teaspoon chilli powder
1 large handful of fresh parsley, chopped
2 tablespoons olive oil

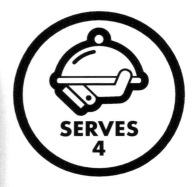

SERVES 4

Method

Heat the olive oil in a pan, add the onion, mushrooms and garlic and cook for 2 minutes until the vegetables have softened. Add the tomatoes, celery, chilli and parsley to the pan with the mushrooms and let it simmer. In the meantime, boil the spaghetti in salted water until cooked through. When the spaghetti is cooked toss it in the tomato and mushroom mixture and serve with an extra sprinkling of parsley.

Broccoli & Cauliflower Fritters

SERVES 2

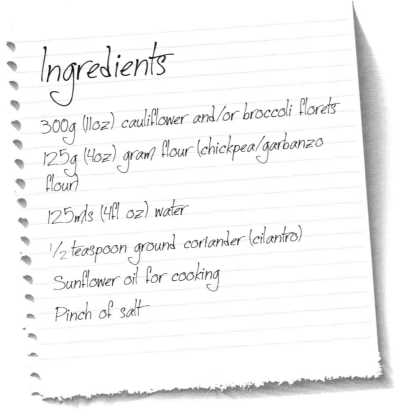

Ingredients

300g (1loz) cauliflower and/or broccoli florets

125g (4oz) gram flour (chickpea/garbanzo flour)

125mls (4fl oz) water

1/2 teaspoon ground coriander (cilantro)

Sunflower oil for cooking

Pinch of salt

Method

Place the flour, salt and ground coriander (cilantro) into a bowl and mix well. Add the water and whisk to a smooth batter. Heat the sunflower oil in a large frying pan. Coat the vegetables in the batter and cook it in the frying pan until golden. Turn it over and cook on the other side. Serve with salad, rice or just with dips like sweet chilli sauce.

Smoky Bean Casserole

Ingredients

400g (14oz) haricot beans, drained and rinsed
400g (14oz) pinto beans, drained and rinsed
400g (14oz) tinned tomatoes, chopped
225g (8oz) button mushrooms, halved
3 garlic cloves, chopped
1 onion, chopped
1 tablespoon smoked paprika
1 teaspoon chilli powder
1 large handful of fresh coriander (cilantro)
250mls (8fl oz) hot vegetable stock (broth)
1 tablespoon olive oil

SERVES
4

Method

Heat the oil in a saucepan, add the onions, mushrooms, garlic, chilli, haricot beans, pinto beans, tomatoes and paprika and cook for 3 minutes. Pour in the stock (broth) and simmer for around 8 minutes or until the vegetables have softened. Stir in the fresh herbs and serve on its own or with rice, quinoa or potatoes.

Vegetable Saute

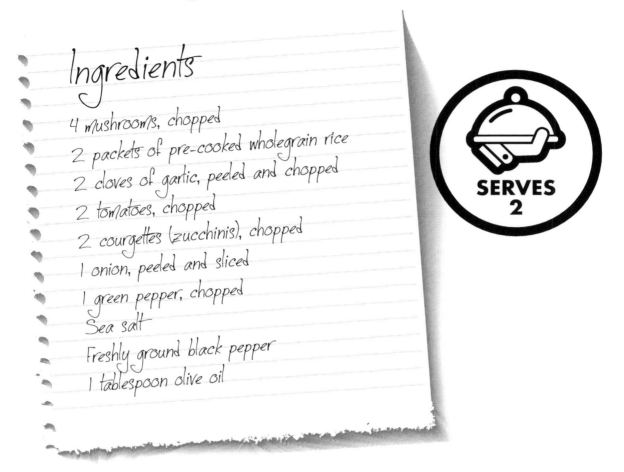

Ingredients

4 mushrooms, chopped

2 packets of pre-cooked wholegrain rice

2 cloves of garlic, peeled and chopped

2 tomatoes, chopped

2 courgettes (zucchinis), chopped

1 onion, peeled and sliced

1 green pepper, chopped

Sea salt

Freshly ground black pepper

1 tablespoon olive oil

SERVES 2

Method

Heat oil in a saucepan, add the onion, mushrooms and garlic and cook for 3 minutes. Add in the courgette (zucchini), green pepper (bell pepper) and tomatoes. Season with salt and pepper. Cook for 5 minutes. In the meantime, warm the rice according to the instructions. Add the rice to the saucepan and stir well. Serve and enjoy.

Barbecued Mushrooms

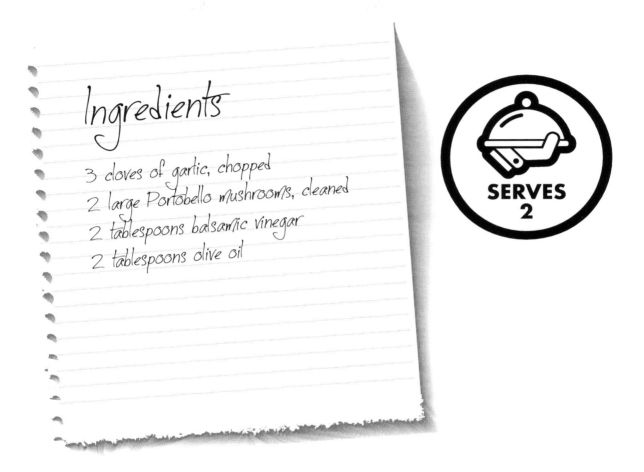

Ingredients

3 cloves of garlic, chopped
2 large Portobello mushrooms, cleaned
2 tablespoons balsamic vinegar
2 tablespoons olive oil

SERVES 2

Method

Remove the mushrooms stalks, chop them and place them in a bowl. Lay the mushrooms with the gills facing up. Place the garlic, balsamic vinegar and olive oil in a bowl and mix well. Spoon the mixture into the mushroom cap. Cook them on a barbecue for 8-10 minutes. Serve with couscous, quinoa, rice or salad.

Chilli & Sesame Quinoa Salad

SERVES 4

Ingredients

- 300g (11oz) quinoa
- 150g (5oz) frozen peas
- 5 radishes, chopped
- 1 large carrot, grated (shredded)
- 1 red pepper (bell pepper) chopped
- 1/2 cucumber, diced
- Handful of cashew nuts

FOR THE DRESSING:

- 1cm (1/2 inch) chunk of fresh ginger, grated (shredded)
- 1/2 -1 teaspoon chilli flakes (or according to taste)
- 3 tablespoons soy sauce
- 1 tablespoon olive oil
- 1 tablespoon sesame oil

Method

Boil the quinoa for around 12 minutes or until the grains have opened and then drain it. Alternatively you can use pre-cooked quinoa to save you time. Cook the peas in boiling water for 2-3 minutes or until heated through, then drain them. Combine all of the vegetables and nuts in a large bowl and stir in the quinoa. In separate bowl mix together the ingredients for the dressing. Pour the dressing onto the salad and mix well.

Lentil & Vegetable Curry

Ingredients

400g (14oz) tin cooked green lentils, rinsed and drained

400g (14oz) tin chopped tomatoes

1 onion, finely chopped

1 clove garlic, finely chopped

1 green pepper (bell pepper), finely chopped

1 tablespoon garam masala

1 teaspoons ground cumin

1 teaspoon ground turmeric

1 tablespoon curry powder

Fresh coriander (cilantro) to garnish (optional)

1 tablespoon olive oil

SERVES 2-3

Method

Heat the oil in a frying pan and add the onion, green pepper (bell pepper) and garlic and cook for 2 minutes. Add in the cumin, garam masala, turmeric and curry powder and mix well. Add in the tomatoes and lentils and cook for 5 minutes. Serve with rice and a sprinkle of coriander (cilantro).

DESSERTS & SNACKS

Fresh Banana Flapjacks

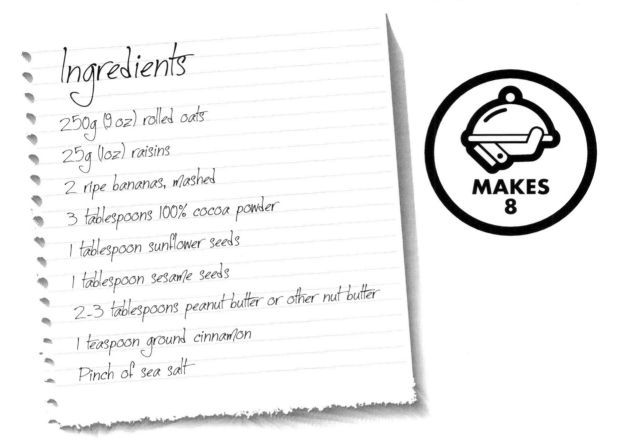

Ingredients

250g (9 oz) rolled oats

25g (1oz) raisins

2 ripe bananas, mashed

3 tablespoons 100% cocoa powder

1 tablespoon sunflower seeds

1 tablespoon sesame seeds

2-3 tablespoons peanut butter or other nut butter

1 teaspoon ground cinnamon

Pinch of sea salt

MAKES 8

Method

Place all of the ingredients into a large bowl and combine them thoroughly. Spoon the oat mixture into a shallow rectangular baking tin. Smooth the mixture out. Place it in the fridge until ready to eat. Cut it into slices and enjoy straight away. You can experiment with different nuts, seeds and dried fruit to find your favourite.

Pistachio & Matcha Energy Balls

Ingredients

200g (7oz) pistachio nuts

100g (3½ oz) dried apricots, chopped

100g (3½ oz) pitted dates

100g (3½ oz) pumpkin seeds

50g (2oz) desiccated (shredded) coconut

2 tablespoons tahini paste

1-2 tablespoons water (optional)

1 teaspoon matcha powder

1 teaspoon maple syrup (optional)

Extra coconut for rolling

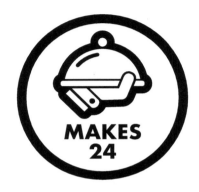

MAKES 24

Method

Place the pistachio nuts, matcha powder, pumpkin seeds and coconut into a food processor and processor until combined. Add in the dates, apricots, tahini and maple syrup (if using). The mixture should be fairly moist but add a tablespoon or two or water if it seems too dry. Using clean hands, roll the mixture into bite-size balls. Scatter the desiccated (shredded) coconut onto a large plate and roll the balls in it. Store in an airtight container, if you don't devour them straight away!

Cranberry & Coconut Truffles

Ingredients

- 100g (3½ oz) oats
- 50g (2oz) desiccated (shredded) coconut
- 50g (2oz) almond or peanut butter
- 50g (2oz) sunflower seeds
- 50g (2oz) dried cranberries
- 2 tablespoons maple syrup
- 3 tablespoons ground linseeds (flaxseeds)
- 1 tablespoon water

Method

Place all of the ingredients in a bowl and mix the ingredients together really well. If the mixture seems to dry add an extra tablespoon of cold water. Using clean hands, roll the mixture into cover it and allow it to sit for 30 minutes, ready to be rolled into bite-size truffles. You can eat them straight away or store them in an airtight container.

Coffee Truffles

Ingredients

275g (10oz) pitted dates

4 tablespoons 100% cocoa powder or cacao nibs

2 tablespoons ground almonds

2 teaspoons cinnamon

2 tablespoons almond butter

3 tablespoons black brewed coffee

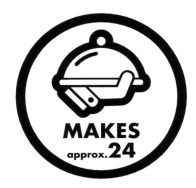

MAKES
approx. **24**

Method

Place all of the ingredients into a blender and blitz until smooth. Using clean hands, shape the mixture into truffles. Store them in an airtight container in the fridge for a tasty energy-boosting snack.

Brazil Nut & Goji Bites

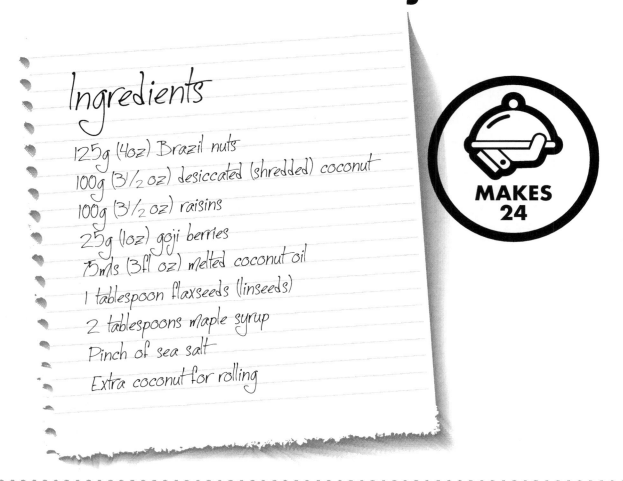

Ingredients

125g (4oz) Brazil nuts

100g (3½ oz) desiccated (shredded) coconut

100g (3½ oz) raisins

25g (1oz) goji berries

75mls (3fl oz) melted coconut oil

1 tablespoon flaxseeds (linseeds)

2 tablespoons maple syrup

Pinch of sea salt

Extra coconut for rolling

MAKES 24

Method

Place all of the ingredients into a food processor and blitz until the mixture is soft. Using clean hands, roll the mixture into balls. Sprinkle some coconut onto a plate and coat the balls in it. Store in an airtight container in the fridge until ready to eat.

Mango Mousse

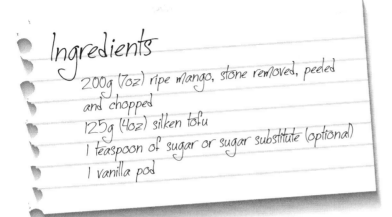

Ingredients

200g (7oz) ripe mango, stone removed, peeled and chopped
125g (4oz) silken tofu
1 teaspoon of sugar or sugar substitute (optional)
1 vanilla pod

SERVES
2

Method

Place the mango, silken tofu, vanilla and sugar (if using) into a blender and process until smooth. Spoon the mousse mixture into bowls. You can eat it straight away or chill before serving.

Strawberry Mousse

Ingredients

200g (7oz) strawberries, hulled and halved
125g (4oz) silken tofu
1 vanilla pod

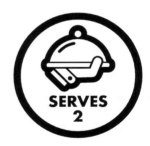

SERVES
2

Method

Place the strawberries in a small pan and simmer for 10-15 minutes or until they are completely soft. Set them aside to cool. Place the strawberries, tofu and vanilla into a blender and process until smooth. Spoon it into glasses or bowls and chill before serving.

Raspberry Crumbles & Coconut Cream

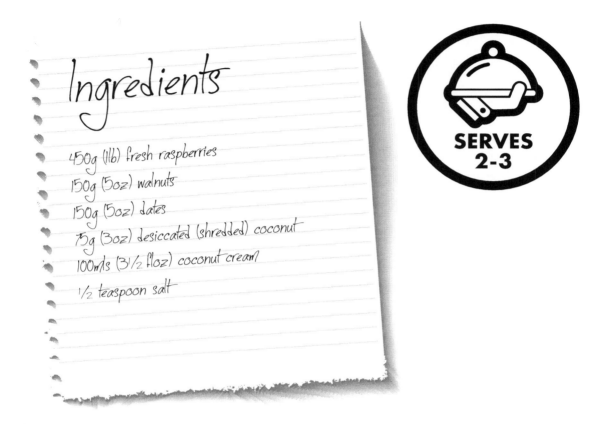

Ingredients

450g (1lb) fresh raspberries

150g (5oz) walnuts

150g (5oz) dates

75g (3oz) desiccated (shredded) coconut

100mls (3½ floz) coconut cream

½ teaspoon salt

SERVES 2-3

Method

Place the walnuts, coconut, dates and salt into a food processor and blitz until it becomes crumbly. Transfer the mixture to a large bowl. Add in the raspberries and mix well. Serve into bowls and add a dollop of coconut cream. Enjoy.

Sweet Sugar-Free Popcorn

SERVES 2

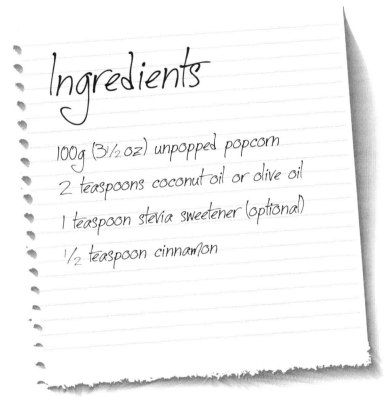

Ingredients

100g (3½ oz) unpopped popcorn

2 teaspoons coconut oil or olive oil

1 teaspoon stevia sweetener (optional)

½ teaspoon cinnamon

Method

Heat the oil and stevia (if using) in a large saucepan and gently warm it while stirring. Add the uncooked popcorn and place a lid on the saucepan. Cook for around 2-3 minutes or until all the corn has popped. Sprinkle on the cinnamon. Allow it to cool before serving.

Dairy-Free Ice Cream

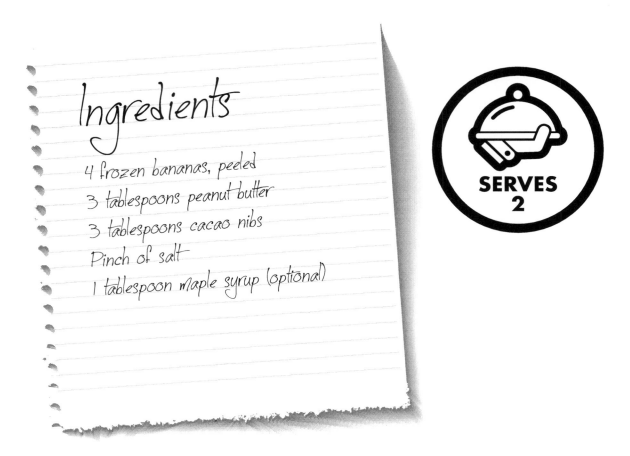

Ingredients

4 frozen bananas, peeled

3 tablespoons peanut butter

3 tablespoons cacao nibs

Pinch of salt

1 tablespoon maple syrup (optional)

SERVES 2

Method

This is a super quick dessert which does require you to freeze some bananas in advance.
Simply put the frozen bananas into a food processor and blitz until they become smooth.
Add in the peanuts butter, cacao nibs, salt and maple syrup (if using) and blend all the
ingredients together. Serve and eat straight away.

Apple & Caramel Dip

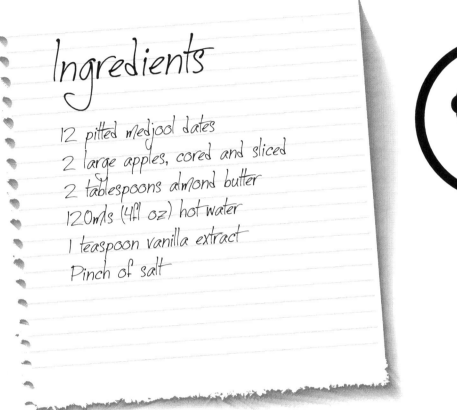

Ingredients

12 pitted medjool dates
2 large apples, cored and sliced
2 tablespoons almond butter
120mls (4fl oz) hot water
1 teaspoon vanilla extract
Pinch of salt

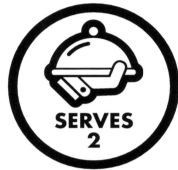

SERVES
2

Method

Place the dates, almond butter, water, vanilla extract and salt into a food processor and combine them until the mixture is smooth and creamy. Spoon the mixture into a small serving bowl. Serve with the apple slices along with the dip.

Turmeric Chai Latte

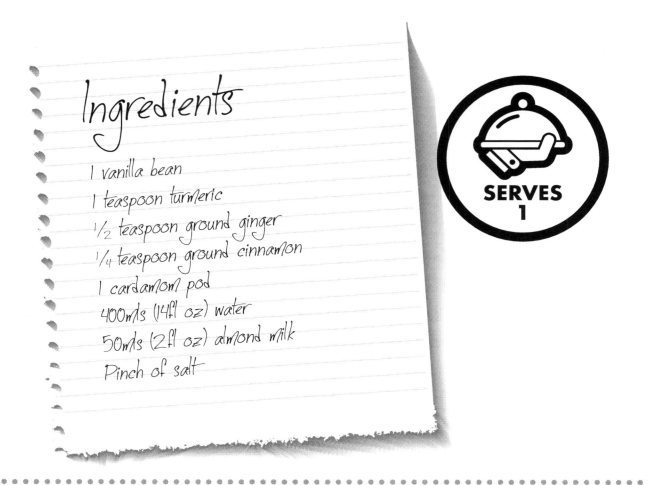

Ingredients

1 vanilla bean
1 teaspoon turmeric
½ teaspoon ground ginger
¼ teaspoon ground cinnamon
1 cardamom pod
400mls (14fl oz) water
50mls (2fl oz) almond milk
Pinch of salt

SERVES 1

Method

Place the cinnamon, ginger, cardamom, vanilla and salt in a saucepan along with the water and bring it to the boil. Reduce the heat and simmer until the mixture reduces to roughly half. In the meantime, heat the almond milk and turmeric in a saucepan, stirring well. Strain the spice liquid through a sieve and pour it into a heat-proof glass. Pour the milk into the glass also and stir. Enjoy.

Pumpkin Pie Spice

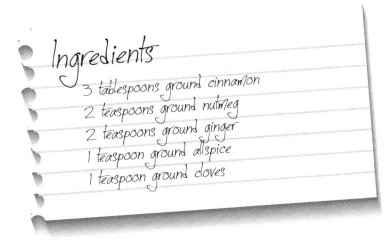

Ingredients

- 3 tablespoons ground cinnamon
- 2 teaspoons ground nutmeg
- 2 teaspoons ground ginger
- 1 teaspoon ground allspice
- 1 teaspoon ground cloves

Method

Mix all of the spices together and store in an airtight container until ready to use.

Pumpkin Spiced Latte

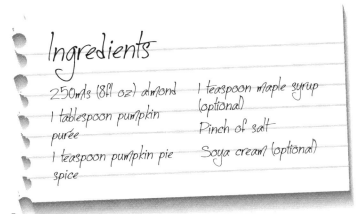

Ingredients

- 250mls (8fl oz) almond
- 1 tablespoon pumpkin purée
- 1 teaspoon pumpkin pie spice
- 1 teaspoon maple syrup (optional)
- Pinch of salt
- Soya cream (optional)

Method

Heat the almond milk in a saucepan (or microwave) and stir in the pumpkin purée and mix well. Pour into your favourite mug. You can add a swirl of soya cream if you wish.

Fruit Infused Water

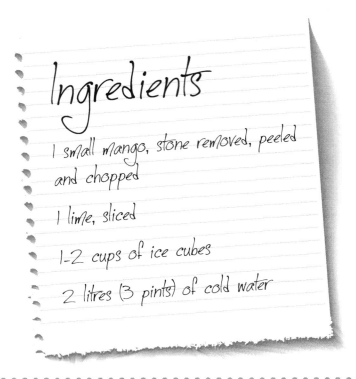

Ingredients

1 small mango, stone removed, peeled and chopped

1 lime, sliced

1-2 cups of ice cubes

2 litres (3 pints) of cold water

Method

Fill a glass jug with water, add the mango, lime and ice. Drink straight away or keep it in the fridge until ready to serve. You can try experimenting with some of the combinations below and find your favourite.

Strawberry & Lime

Cucumber & Fresh Mint

Apple, Ginger & Cinnamon

Apricot & Raspberry

Raspberry & Orange

Pineapple & Mango

Cucumber & Lemon

Lemon & Ginger

Lime & Cucumber

Raspberry & Basil

Orange & Thyme

Pineapple, Cherry & Lemon

Kiwi & Lemon

Cherry Chocolate Milkshake

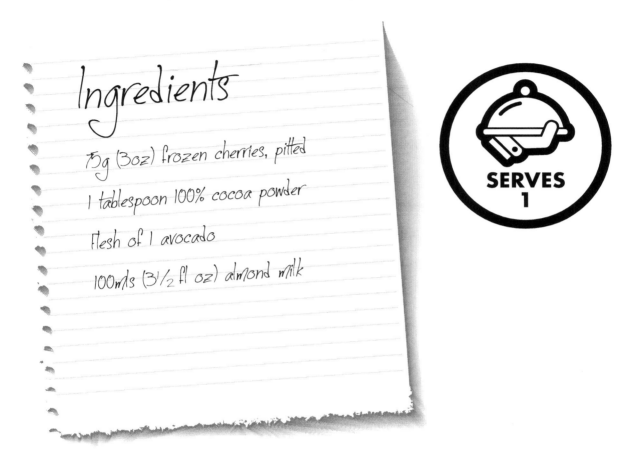

Ingredients

75g (3oz) frozen cherries, pitted

1 tablespoon 100% cocoa powder

Flesh of 1 avocado

100mls (3½ fl oz) almond milk

SERVES 1

Method

Place all of the ingredients into a food processor or smoothie maker and process until smooth and creamy. Serve and enjoy.

DIPS, SAUCES & DRESSINGS

Satay Dressing

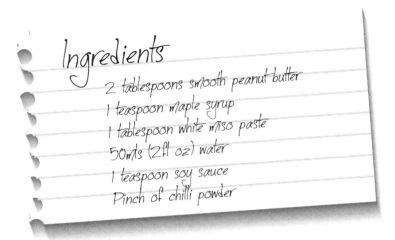

Ingredients

2 tablespoons smooth peanut butter
1 teaspoon maple syrup
1 tablespoon white miso paste
50mls (2fl oz) water
1 teaspoon soy sauce
Pinch of chilli powder

Method

Place all of the ingredients into a bowl and mix well.

Creamy Tahini Dressing

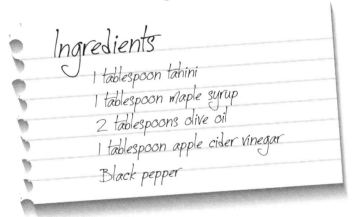

Ingredients

1 tablespoon tahini
1 tablespoon maple syrup
2 tablespoons olive oil
1 tablespoon apple cider vinegar
Black pepper

SERVES
2

Method

Combine all of the ingredients in a bowl and season with pepper.

Lemon, Basil & Walnut Dressing

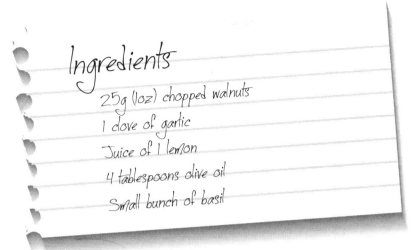

Ingredients

- 25g (1oz) chopped walnuts
- 1 clove of garlic
- Juice of 1 lemon
- 4 tablespoons olive oil
- Small bunch of basil

Method

Place all the ingredients into a blender and blitz until smooth.

Coriander & Lime Dressing

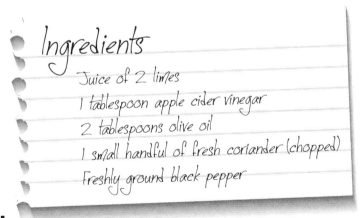

Ingredients

- Juice of 2 limes
- 1 tablespoon apple cider vinegar
- 2 tablespoons olive oil
- 1 small handful of fresh coriander (chopped)
- Freshly ground black pepper

Method

Place all of the ingredients into a food processor and blitz until smooth. Serve it with beans, rice and salads.

Sweet Chilli Dressing

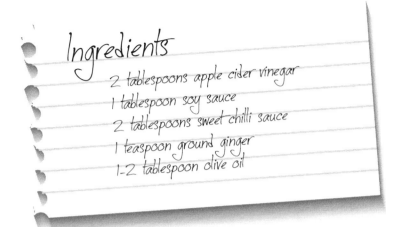

Ingredients

2 tablespoons apple cider vinegar
1 tablespoon soy sauce
2 tablespoons sweet chilli sauce
1 teaspoon ground ginger
1-2 tablespoon olive oil

SERVES
2-3

Method

Combine all of the ingredients in a bowl and mix well. Serve with tofu dishes, Buddha bowls and salads.

Curry Dressing

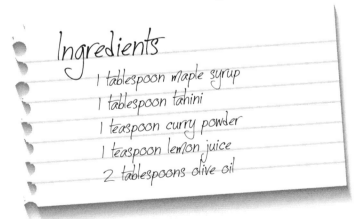

Ingredients

1 tablespoon maple syrup
1 tablespoon tahini
1 teaspoon curry powder
1 teaspoon lemon juice
2 tablespoons olive oil

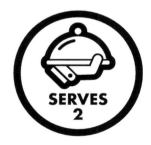

SERVES
2

Method

Place all of the ingredients into a bowl and mix well. Serve with bean dishes and salads.

Basic Vinaigrette

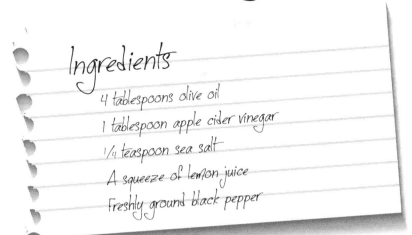

Ingredients

- 4 tablespoons olive oil
- 1 tablespoon apple cider vinegar
- 1/4 teaspoon sea salt
- A squeeze of lemon juice
- Freshly ground black pepper

Method

Place all of the ingredients into a bowl or jar and mix well. You can add a clove of garlic, fresh or dried herbs, or a teaspoon of mustard or balsamic to this basic mixture for extra flavour.

Tropical Dressing

Ingredients

- 1 avocado, stone removed and peeled
- 1 tablespoon tahini
- 75mls (2fl oz) orange juice
- 50mls (2fl oz) pineapple juice
- 2 tablespoons olive oil or avocado oil
- 2 teaspoons soy sauce
- Pinch of cayenne pepper
- Freshly ground black pepper

Method

Place all of the ingredients into a blender and blitz until smooth and creamy. If the dressing seems to think you can add a little extra juice or oil.

Mediterranean Dressing

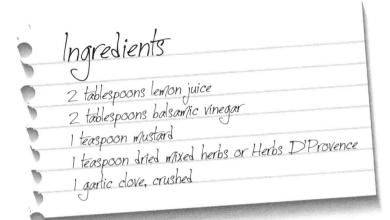

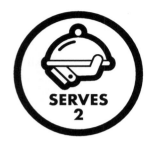

SERVES 2

Ingredients

2 tablespoons lemon juice
2 tablespoons balsamic vinegar
1 teaspoon mustard
1 teaspoon dried mixed herbs or Herbs D'Provence
1 garlic clove, crushed

Method

Place all the ingredients together in a bowl and mix well. Use this dressing in Buddha bowls and salads. It's such a versatile dressing so it may be helpful to increase the quantities in the store it in an airtight container in the fridge for a day or two.

Peanut, Ginger & Lime Dressing

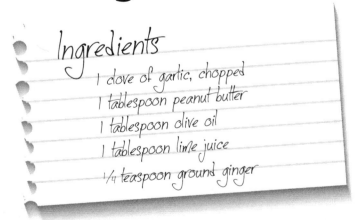

Ingredients

1 clove of garlic, chopped
1 tablespoon peanut butter
1 tablespoon olive oil
1 tablespoon lime juice
1/4 teaspoon ground ginger

Method

Place all the ingredients into a bowl and mix well.

Avocado & Basil Dressing

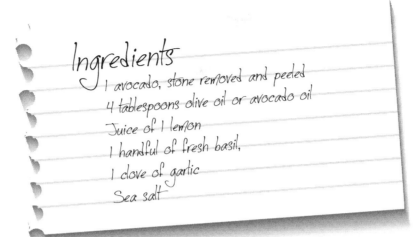

Ingredients
1 avocado, stone removed and peeled
4 tablespoons olive oil or avocado oil
Juice of 1 lemon
1 handful of fresh basil,
1 clove of garlic
Sea salt

Method

Place all of the ingredients into a food processor and blitz until smooth and creamy. Use straight away.

Sweet Orange & Mustard Dressing

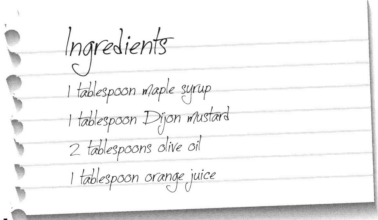

Ingredients
1 tablespoon maple syrup
1 tablespoon Dijon mustard
2 tablespoons olive oil
1 tablespoon orange juice

Method

Place all of the ingredients into a bowl and mix well. This is delicious with heaps of green salad and pine nuts.

Smoky Tomato Dip

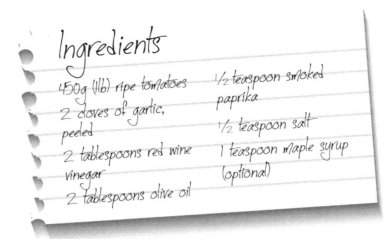

Ingredients

450g (1lb) ripe tomatoes

2 cloves of garlic, peeled

2 tablespoons red wine vinegar

2 tablespoons olive oil

½ teaspoon smoked paprika

½ teaspoon salt

1 teaspoon maple syrup (optional)

Method

Place all of the ingredients into a blender and blitz until smooth. Use as a dip or add a spoonful to salads.

Cheese-Free Pesto

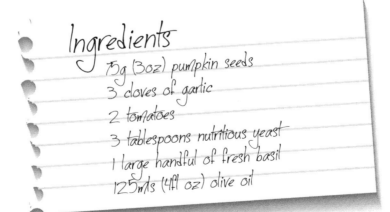

Ingredients

75g (3oz) pumpkin seeds

3 cloves of garlic

2 tomatoes

3 tablespoons nutritious yeast

1 large handful of fresh basil

125mls (4fl oz) olive oil

Method

Place all of the ingredients, except the oil, into a blender and blitz until well combined. Slowly add the oil and blend it as you go until the mixture is smooth.

Barbecue Sauce

Ingredients

150g (5oz) tomato purée (paste)

2 tablespoons mustard

2 tablespoons smoked paprika

1 tablespoon garlic powder

1 teaspoon sea salt

2 teaspoons black pepper

1 teaspoon sugar (optional)

150mls (5fl oz) apple cider vinegar

3-4 tablespoons maple syrup

Method

Combine all of the ingredients until mixed well. Can be used hot or cold. Use it as a marinade for tofu and vegetables or warm the sauce over a medium heat and serve it with chips, sweet potato fries or burgers.

Vegan 'Parmesan' Cheese

Ingredients

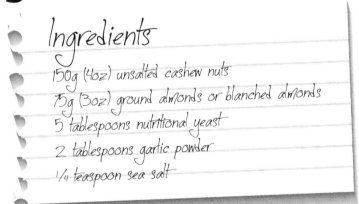

150g (4oz) unsalted cashew nuts

75g (3oz) ground almonds or blanched almonds

5 tablespoons nutritional yeast

2 tablespoons garlic powder

1/4 teaspoon sea salt

Method

Place all of the ingredients into a food processor and blend until the mixture is fine and crumbly, like Parmesan cheese. Use it straight away or store it in an airtight container in the fridge until ready to use.

Vegan Mayonnaise

Ingredients

350g (12oz) silken tofu, drained
3 tablespoons lemon juice
1/2 teaspoon mustard
1/2 teaspoon sea salt
2 teaspoons olive oil

Method

Place the tofu into a food processor and blitz until it's completely smooth. Add in the lemon juice, salt, mustard and olive oil and combine the ingredients. Transfer the mayonnaise to jar or airtight container and keep refrigerated. You can also add a clove or two of chopped garlic to make garlic mayonnaise.

Guacamole

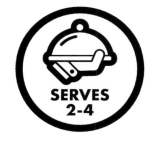

SERVES
2-4

Ingredients

2 ripe avocados
1 clove garlic
1 red chilli pepper, finely chopped
Juice of 1/2 lime

Method

Remove the stone from the avocados and scoop out the flesh. Place all the ingredients in a bowl and mash together until smooth or alternatively use a food processor. Serve with crackers, toast, loaded potatoes, with raw crudités or as a sandwich filler.

Hummus

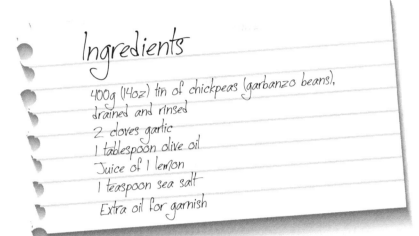

Ingredients

400g (14oz) tin of chickpeas (garbanzo beans),
drained and rinsed
2 cloves garlic
1 tablespoon olive oil
Juice of 1 lemon
1 teaspoon sea salt
Extra oil for garnish

Method

Place all the ingredients in a food processor and mix until smooth and creamy. Transfer it to a bowl and add a little swirl of olive oil on top.

Beetroot Hummus

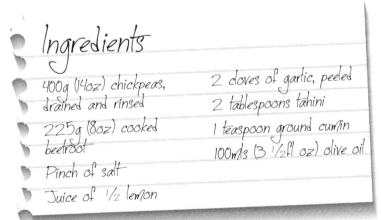

Ingredients

400g (14oz) chickpeas,
drained and rinsed
225g (8oz) cooked
beetroot
Pinch of salt
Juice of ½ lemon

2 cloves of garlic, peeled
2 tablespoons tahini
1 teaspoon ground cumin
100mls (3 ½fl oz) olive oil

Method

Place all of the ingredients into a blender and blitz until smooth. Serve as a dip or in Buddha bowls and salads.

You may also be interested in other titles by
Erin Rose Publishing
which are available in both paperback and ebook.

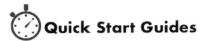 Quick Start Guides

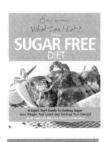 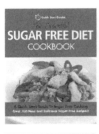 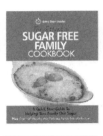 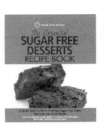 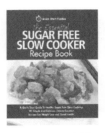 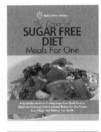

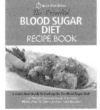 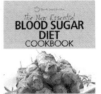 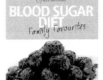 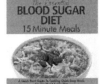 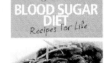

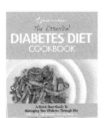 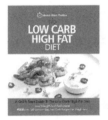 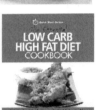 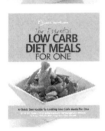 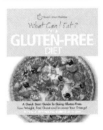 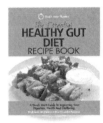

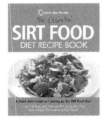 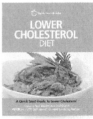 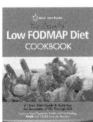 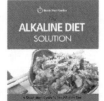 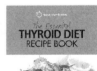

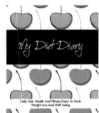 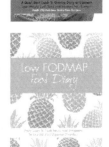 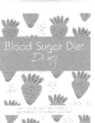 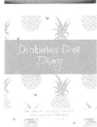 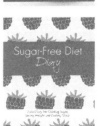 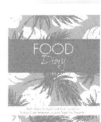

Books by Sophie Ryan
Erin Rose Publishing

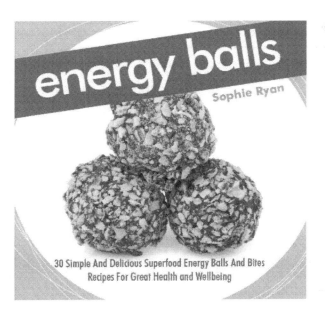

30 Simple And Delicious Superfood Energy Balls And Bites
Recipes For Great Health and Wellbeing

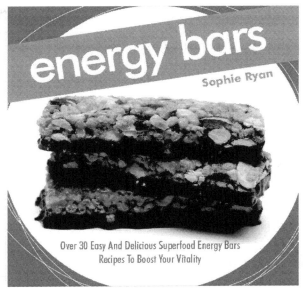

Over 30 Easy And Delicious Superfood Energy Bars
Recipes To Boost Your Vitality

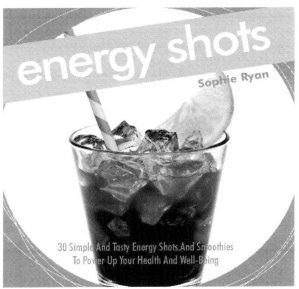

30 Simple And Tasty Energy Shots And Smoothies
To Power Up Your Health And Well-Being

Printed in Great Britain
by Amazon